Mind-Body-Soul Aromatherapy

Mind-Body-Soul Aromatherapy

Heidi Murphy, M. Ed.

D. S. Murphy, N.D.

The first edition of this book was titled *An Introduction to the Art of Aromatherapy*.

ISBN-13: 978-1482608991

ISBN-10: 1482608995

Bound and printed in the United States of America by CreateSpace, an Amazon company.

Dr. Dave is also the author of Compass Wellness Coaching: 360 Degree Wellness Coaching

---

This book is intended to be educational and as a reference volume only but not as a medical manual. The information given in this book is designed to help you help others make informed decisions about total wellness. This book is not intended as a substitute for any treatment that has been or may be prescribed by your doctor, or the doctors of your clients. If you suspect that you or one of your clients has a medical problem then I urge you to seek competent medical help from a licensed medical practitioner. Aromatherapists are not licensed medical practitioners and do not diagnose or treat medical conditions.

For our boys

Geoffrey

Ernest and

Brandon

Contents

Introduction

Welcome to the exciting and rewarding world of aromatherapy. Aromatherapy is the smell of life. The essential oils used in aromatherapy capture the natural essences of plants and flowers, the product of biochemical reactions and sunlight. The biochemical complexities essential oils are hard to capture in traditional pharmaceuticals as are the complex interactions of essential oils with the human body. Thus aromatherapy is an art more than a science. You will learn through practice and experience what works best.

Aromatherapy is, of all the alternative medicine protocols the most accessible, and the most enjoyable. Learning how to use essential oils to improve the quality of your life or those of others is not a daunting task. And what could be more enjoyable than experimenting with the different aromas of beautiful plants and flowers.

This book begins with a short introduction to aromatherapy and the history or evolution of the art. While you may never want to produce essential oils it is important to understand how they are produced and especially how to care for your essential oils to preserve their healing qualities. Chapter Five provides an overview of how essential oils interact with the human body, but through massage and through inhalation. Chapter Six is the heart of the book. This chapter will provide with you an in-depth understand of the uses and effects of some of the most important essential oils. Most essential oils are too strong to use used neat (full strength) so Chapter Seven gives you an overview of common carrier oils used with essential oils. Chapter Eight explains how to blend essential oils for different uses and Chapter Nine gives you some ideas in case you are interested in starting an aromatherapy business.

The resource section at the end of the book lists essential oil suppliers, bottle suppliers and professional associations for aromatherapists.

One

Introduction to Aromatherapy

Welcome to the exciting world of aromtherapy. More than one-third of Americans use alternative medical treatments for serious medical conditions every year spending over $14 billion in the process. Aromatherapy is one of the many alternative treatments that have become popular.

Aromatherapy is the use of the natural plant essences to improve the health and wellbeing of the body, mind and spirit (emotions). It is not just a beauty treatment or a simple relaxation method. Essential plant oils are capable of restoring the body's harmony and equilibrium. The selection of the appropriate essential oils is more of a creative art than a science and consequently aromatherapy is one of the true healing art.

Some aromatherapists practice *clinical or medical aromatherapy*. They use essential oils to treat specific medical conditions, often under the direction and supervision of a physician or other health care professional, according to the principles of traditional Western medical theories and practices. Medical aromatherapy does not always include the application of essential oils by massage, many other methods of administration are also used. Medical aromatherapy is most commonly used in France.

Holistic aromatherapy is related to medical aromatherapy but is used by practitioners of holistic or alternative medicine. Holistic aromatherapy is used to promote and maintain health and well-being. Usually the practitioners consult with their patient so that they can select the most appropriate essential oils. Massage techniques are often used to apply the selected essential oils. Massage therapists, naturopathic physicians, other natural health practitioners often use holistic aromatherapy.

The use of essential oils as an enhanced skin care technique is called *aesthetic aromatherapy*. Essential oils can be added to skin care products or applied directly to the skin with a base or carrier oil. You may have thought about preparing your own personal face cream and including one or more essential oils in the formulation.

Because essential oils can have a profound effect on emotions and the mind they are sometimes used in *psycho-aromatherapy*. Essential oils can be used a stimulants, as sedatives or as regulators or moderators of mental and emotional functions. In the following pages we will review research in this area that has been conducted in both the United States and England.

You may be interested in one of these uses of aromatherapy or you may plan on using aromatherapy in your home to treat yourself and your family and friends. It doesn't matter what your plans are, aromatherapy is an exciting and rewarding and very effective.

One of the most fascinating aspects of aromatherapy is the effect of aromas on the mind and the emotions. Your sense of smell is the most sensitive of your five senses. The sense of smell is activated by only eight aroma molecules and only forty molecules are needed to be able to recognize a specific aroma. Most people can detect a single bell pepper molecule in a trillion molecules of air. These molecules enter your nasal cavity where they are detected by about ten million smell receptors. The receptors are covered by *olfactory cilia* that look like small hair fibers that move back and forth on the air currents. You have about twenty million cilia clustered around the ten million neurons in your olfactory system. According to one theory, each receptor functions as the key to a specific odor and that this key "unlocks" the identification of the specific odor. Each receptor is connected to the brain by an *olfactory nerve*.

Figure 1
Sense of Smell

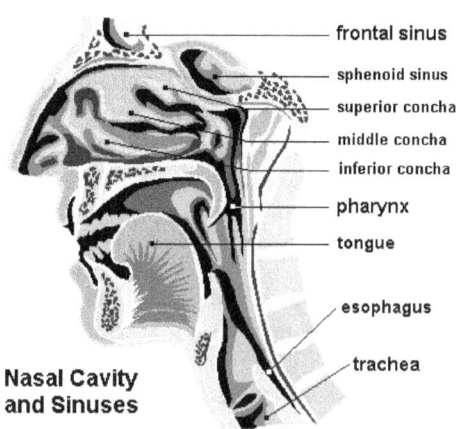

frontal sinus
sphenoid sinus
superior concha
middle concha
inferior concha
pharynx
tongue
esophagus
trachea

Nasal Cavity and Sinuses

The sense of smell is the only one of your five senses in which the corresponding nerves are connected directly to the brain. This is why some say that the practice of aromatherapy is really the practice of psycho-aromatherapy. Figure 1 above depicts the components of your upper respiratory system.

What can aromatherapy do for you?

Nature has provided you with essential oils that have valuable healing properties. When highly concentrated these essential oils are ideal for treating a diversity of physical, mental and emotional ills. Aromatherapy works on the body in a very natural and holistic way. Essential oils gently activate the healing energy of your body to help it restore its emotional, mental and physical equilibrium. Aromatherapy can be used in conjunction with any of the healing arts, both conventional and alternative.

Aromatherapy is a simple way of improving the quality of your health and life and of your family members and friends. In general it helps your mind and body work more efficiently and it has the capacity to reinforce your auto-immune system. In addition, aromatherapy can help you reduce the effects of stress in your life and have a positive influence on your emotions. Many of the essential oils help regulate your sense of well-being. Some essential oils work as central nervous system energizers and stimulants, others work as sedatives and tranquilizers, others restore emotional and mental equilibrium.

You can add a new dimension to you skin and hair care programs with aromatherapy too. Aromatherapy is one of the most natural and effective beauty treatments known. Essential oils will give your skin and hair a healthy appearance. Various essential oils can be used to revitalize dry or prematurely aged skin, control oily skin, and to treat skin diseases. The specific effects of different essential oils and their uses are presented in Chapters 6 and 7.

Aromatherapy and Alternative Medicine

You may not realize it, but as a practitioner of aromatherapy you are also practicing alternative or holistic medicine. The basic philosophy of holistic medicine is to treat the person and not the disease. Modern or conventional medicine (allopathic medicine) is the study and treatment of disease. Alternative or holistic medicine (naturopathy) is the study and maintenance of health. Naturopathy treats a sick person, not a sick organ. Conventional medicine uses drugs, radiation, surgery and other invasive procedures in its war on disease. Naturopathic medicine on the other hand uses nutrition, herbs, reflexology, iridology, clinical kinesiology, massage and other noninvasive procedures to help a body reach and maintain internal harmony or homeostasis. Aromatherapy is one way in which an alternative medicine practitioner makes use of herbs in treatments.

Hypocrites reminded physicians in his oath to "First, do no harm". The philosophy of holistic medicine is in keeping with this injunction. Conventional medicine, while necessary, may damage the body while fighting disease. For example, antibiotics may be prescribed to fight a bacterial infection. Unfortunately antibiotics are not bacteria specific; they are "broad spectrum" drugs. This means that the antibiotics kill not just the bad bacteria that has infected a person but all bacteria, including good bacteria that aid digestion.

Another difference between conventional medicine and holistic medicine is the philosophy of disease. Diseases, according to conventional medicine, are caused by external pathogens like bacteria. These diseases can be identified, named and attacked. Given sufficient time, resources and drugs any disease can thus be conquered. Holistic medicine rejects the bacteriological origin of disease. Its philosophical premise is that microorganisms are not the primary causes of disease but rather lack of harmony (homeostasis) in the body. The lack of harmony may be caused by poorly functioning metabolism or organic malfunctions that weaken the body and make it susceptible to illness.

To naturopaths there is but one disease, a general state of ill health, which may manifest itself in different forms. The manifestation appears in the "weak link" in a person's chain of health. The weak link may result from normal genetic predispositions, autointoxication, enervation (deprivation or diminution of nerve force or energy), nutritional deficiencies and/or immunological deficiencies. The local manifestation of illness is symptomatic of a systemic problem that usually requires both local and systemic treatment. Aromatherapy, the use of concentrated herbal extracts, is both a systemic and local treatment. As a systemic treatment, aromatherapy affects the physical, emotional, mental and spiritual states and helps a person achieve harmony.

We have talked a little about harmony. A more technical term is homeostasis. It is the condition in which body systems are maintained at their optimal levels. Your body constantly tries to maintain harmony or homeostasis, and when it does you are a living organism that is functioning properly. This auto regulation is controlled by the endocrine and autonomic nervous systems. However, your internal harmony is affected by internal and external factors like your diet, rest and drinking habits, physical and/or emotional stress, drug (prescription and other) related toxins, environmental pollution and toxins and additives in the food that you eat. Conventional medicine makes extensive use of drug therapy. Although well-intentioned and sometimes necessary, drugs disturb homeostasis. Essential oils help restore homeostasis rather than disturb it because they are natural substances.

Two

History of Aromatherapy

The Ancient World

The term "aromatherapy" was coined by the French Chemist René Gattefossé in the 1920s. However, the use of essential oils has a much longer history. More than three thousand years ago the Egyptians used infusions of cedar wood and myrrh to embalm the rich. They used less expensive infusions of cinnamon, elm, sandalwood and thyme to preserve the remains of the common folk.

Archeologists think that the Egyptians, rather than using essential oils, used plant and plant-gum infusions. According to their theories, the Egyptians placed the vegetable matter in containers filled with oil or grease and left the containers out under the hot sun for a few days until the oil was impregnated with aroma. There is also evidence that they obtained essential oils from some plants by placing the plant material in long pieces of cloth and then wringing the cloth to squeeze the oil out of the vegetable matter. The favorite incense in the Egyptian temples was *kyphi*, an aphrodisiac made of about fifteen different ingredients including saffron, drumstick tree, spikenard, cinnamon and Juniper.

At about the same time Ayurvedic medicine was being developed in India. The *Vedas*, sacred books of the Hindu, mention the therapeutic properties of aromatic plants like cilantro, ginger, myrrh, sandalwood and rose. The *Kamasutra* suggests the use of sandalwood as an aphrodisiac and for use in cosmetics.

The Babylonian Empire was one of the principal sources and users of essential oils in the ancient world. They used enormous quantities of silver fir, cedar wood, cypress, juniper, myrrh, pine and rose. Only the rich in Egypt could afford to use perfumes. In ancient Babylon all of the citizens were required by law to use perfume, probably to mask their body odors.

Aromatic substances were also in use in this epoch in the Orient. The ancient Chinese and Japanese used perfumes in the religious ceremonies. Aromatic herbs and woods were used in their funeral rites. Mo-lu-hwa, a variety of Jasmine, was used in China in ancestor veneration ceremonies. Other aromatic herbs were used in conjunction with massage and acupuncture. For example, well-to-do

Chinese families burned Artemis' salt to attract spirits which would ensure that delivery was easy and successful.

Greece and Rome

The Greeks' knowledge of aromatic plant substances, medicine and anatomy was based on the developments of the Egyptians. As in Egypt, the use of aromatic plants was part of the Greek life style. Aphrodite, the goddess of love in Greek mythology, caused perfume to rain down from heaven upon the inhabitants of the earth. Plants were of divine origin for the ancient Greeks and consequently plants had spiritual qualities. In Greece aromatic plant extracts were not used just to perfume bodies and clothing, but also food and wine.

Like the aromatherapists of today, the ancient Greeks recognized that plant aromas not only have therapeutic and medicinal value in treating the body but that they can also be used to treat emotional and nervous problems. They believed that aromas had the power to restore physical health and to heal the mind. Hippocrates taught that a daily aromatic bath followed by a massage with natural perfumes had the power to prolong life. They felt that massage was so effective that Plato scolded Heredities, one of Hippocrates' teachers, for using it to prolonging the miserable lives of the old.

The Romans inherited their knowledge of the uses of aromatic plants from the Greeks. Aromatic substances were used by the Romans in cosmetics, and for personal hygiene, therapy and massages. We all have heard about the public baths in ancient Rome. These baths were an important ritual in Rome. Aromatic oils were added to the steam baths. It was customary to end the baths with a massage and of course aromatic massage oils were used. The use of aromatic substances was not restricted to the bath houses in Rome. Aromas were also used as perfumes for bodies and clothing, homes and even in governmental ceremonies.

Middle Ages

With the collapse of the Roman Empire in the fifth century Roman knowledge and influence disappeared almost completely from Europe. Unfortunately the Western world lost most of its knowledge of the therapeutic, medicinal and cosmetic uses of aromatic plants. All was not lost because the Arabs continued to research, use and export plant-based perfumes. For example, their doctors used sandalwood, camphor, and rose as disinfectants. They also used essential oils to perfume the rooms of the sick, a practice that had been taught by Hippocrates.

In the eleventh century Avicenna (Abu Ibn Sina), the famous Arab doctor, philosopher, mathematician, and astronomer, perfected the distillation process that is still in use today to obtain the volatile oils from plants. He also used massages and a fruit-based detoxification diet as part of his healing process.

The Renaissance to the Modern Era

Perfumers rose to prominence and increased in number during the second half of the Sixteenth Century. During this period people thought that bathing was unhealthy and so they once again began to use perfumes to mask their body odors. Juniper, pine and thyme were used throughout Europe to combat illness, especially the plague, in this era.

It is interesting to note that during the reign of Henry III of France (1551-1589) the use of perfumes became extravagant. The French not only perfumed their bodies and clothing but also their hair, homes, paper and envelops, water, wine and even public fountains.

The religious climate in Europe changed during the sixteenth and seventeenth centuries. This was the time of the Puritans in England and the Spanish Inquisition. The use of perfumes diminished with the changes in the social climate. By the eighteenth century those with strong Puritan beliefs stopped using perfumes and cosmetics. Many in England thought that perfumes and cosmetics were a form of witchcraft that gave women the power to seduce men, causing them to loose control of their senses. Like-minded politicians proposed a law that would have prohibited the use of fragrances.

Scientific advances in the nineteenth century, especially in the field of organic chemistry, resulted in a further decline in the use of natural plan extracts. The perfume industry began to replace natural plant oils with synthetic substitutes because, like today, they were less expensive. Consequently perfumes lost their natural components and therapeutic benefits. Today only the most expensive perfumes contain even infinitesimal quantities of pure plant essences.

The Present

The rebirth of the use of natural essential oils happened by accident in the 1920s. The French chemist and perfumist, René-Maurice Gattefossé was working in his laboratory when he suffered a serious burn on his hand. Acting rapidly, he immersed his hand in the closest container full of a liquid. The container happened to be full of Lavender oil. He noted some time later that his hand had healed very rapidly and without scaring. Because of that fortunate result he dedicated the rest of his life to the study of the therapeutic properties of essential oils. His influence is also the reason for the extensive use today of essential oils by physicians in France. Interest around the world in the values of essential oils has continued to grow among those interested in natural health and holistic healing.

Today two of the most important organizations for practicing aromatherapists are the *National Association for Holistic Aromatherapy* in the United States (www.naha.org) and *The International Federation of Professional Aromatherapists* (http://ifparoma.org/) located in Great Britain. You should contact one of these organizations if you plan on practicing aromatherapy.

Three
Spiritual Healing

Aromatic herbs and incenses have been used in special ceremonies and rituals in many ancient traditions. Many Egyptians, Greek and Roman cultures used aromatherapy. Throughout the centuries aromatherapy has been used both as a means for purification, to summon gods and goddesses, and for energy healing.

It seems that the ancient Greeks honored their priests and priestesses, who were very knowledgeable about blending essences and fragrances to heal body and the soul. They used fragrances in many of their rituals, especially to worship the goddesses Aphrodite and Diana. Their wisdom and knowledge of aromatherapy and plant consciousness were very advanced and it is reported that they used special fragrance sachet of magnolia under their pillows to help them sleep.

Many priests, who acted as representatives of the gods, received instructions about how to make specific herbal combinations to bring healing and spiritual purification to their followers. Because ancient societies had no comprehensible explanations for how plants healed, spiritual groups were formed and supernatural explanations were given to the powerful healing properties of plants and herbs.

Aromatherapy oils were used in magic practice for their vibrations or essences. Aromatherapy oils were sacred to a god or goddess. If we look at different magical traditions or different practitioners of magic or witchcraft we find that they made extensive use of herbs, potions with essential oils. Often these substances were used dedicate and bless themselves before rituals. They also used essential oils to dedicate their ritual instruments and to connect them to the magical realm of nature.

Today aromatherapy oils and extracts are used in ceremonial magic to invoke the energy of a particular deity or goddess. Oils are often used to define the boundaries of a sacred space. The use of vaporizer is a small ritual in itself, as it contains the four elements: air, in which the oils are vaporized, fire, which heats the element of water in which the oils are dispersed and earth, in which the plants are grown. This is an example in how powerful aromatherapy is and how symbolic it can become.

The Earth Connection

When one uses aromatherapy one draws healing from Mother Earth. The high vibrational rate of plants and flowers is probably the highest in nature. Earth has secret codes for healing and balance. These earth codes are ideal for many healing rituals from the past and the present. We know now that aromatherapy oils also affect the body's energy system, and auric field.

Many shamans and indigenous cultures use plants and roots to enhance their sacred spaces, they call unseen forces or deities and use different fragrances and roots from plants and trees to connect deeply with their guides. Many Eastern cultures are in touch with Earth. They feel an intense connection and they don't feel separated from Earth like many of us do in Western civilizations. Lifestyles in indigenous cultures revolve around Earth, plants, herbs and self- reliance. Many people from Native American cultures also respect plants and they ask for plant's permission being removing them from the ground as a way of expressing gratitude and asking for blessings. Chants are used for special rituals and ceremonies to connect with Earth and the other elements. It would be wonderful if all of us could understand and appreciate Mother Nature and feel deep connection with the earth that is felt is some cultures. One never wastes time by asking Mother Earth for healing gifts nor for expressing gratitude to Her.

Balancing Chakras with Aromatherapy Essences

Our chakras respond to the energetic frequencies of our human energy field, known as the body of light. Our chakras are receptive to emotions of others and our emotions. They are sensitive to our energetic field, and conversely, our energetic field affects how open or closed is our chakras system. Essential oils contribute to increase the frequency of our chakra centers, by expanding, refreshing and activating our cellular and etheric bodies. The essences of flowers carry beautiful aromas that have a positive effect on our brain chemistry and also affect our chakra system in accordance with those changes in mental states.

Table 1 provides a summary of the essential oils that are most appropriate for each particular chakra center.

Table 1

Essential Oils and the Chakras

Chakra	Essential Oils
Root	Myrrh, Patchouli, Cedarwood Sandalwood, Vetiver, and Frankincense
Sacral	Ylang Ylang, Cedarwood, Jasmine, Patchouli, Sandalwood, Cinnamon, and Rose
Solar Plexus	Ylang Ylang, Chamomile, Cypress, and Basil
Heart	Ylang Ylang, Cinnamon, Neroli, Palma Rosa, Lavender, Geranium, Clary Sage, Myrrh, Ginger, and Rose
Throat	Rosewood, Chamomile, Lemongrass, Lemon, Palma Rosa, Jasmine, and Pine
Third Eye	Peppermint, Basil, Rosemary, and Lemongrass
Crown	Frankincense, Cedar wood, Myrrh, Sandalwood and Patchouli

Base Chakra

The base chakra is located in the base of the spine and unlike the other main chakras which point forward, it points downwards and slightly forward. Emotionally and psychologically, the base chakra is concerned with the qualities of order, security and stability, self-preservation, survival and animal strength. It is color is red. The root chakra is the source of our vital energy. Our feelings of safety, security, and courage reside here.

When the base chakra is open and functioning we can overcome our fears and receive what we need from life. We become outgoing, alive and fulfilled.

Sacral Chakra

The sacral chakra is located between the genitals and the naval. Its color is orange. It is concerned with self-gratification, well-being, physical comfort, pleasure and sexuality. From the sacral chakra, we regulate our feelings and our emotional expressions. The sacral chakra also provides our physical body with graceful movement. The sacral chakra is the sphere of desires, physical pleasures and happiness. We are connected to our feelings and our sense of physical balance through this chakra. Pleasure helps us sustain a peaceful and joyful life and diminish the perception of pain and suffering.

When the blockage in this chakra is released there will also be a release of long held-back emotions, and physically the body will move again with fluid gracefulness.

Solar Plexus Chakra

The solar plexus chakra is located between the naval and the sternum. Its color is yellow. It is the energy center concerned with the digestion of experience; taking what is of use from life and casting aside what is redundant. It is also the center of our personal power, our identity, self-expression, fulfillment and completeness. It provides us with energy to reach our full potential and goals. If we know who we are we can be true to ourselves, and our goals and objectives. This chakra helps us maintain our true identity regarding of the opinion of others.

When the solar-plexus chakra is unblocked, there is an immediate sense of self-confidence and all fears of self-expression are released.

Heart Chakra

The heart chakra is located over the heart area and is orientated to self-acceptance and social identity. Its color is green. Developing an open heart chakra center also help us practice compassion and self-healing. It is the center concerned with compassion, love, nurturing, trust, emotions, group consciousness, joy, softness in strength, and empathy. When our heart chakra is open and expanded we cultivate attitudes based on love, understanding and emotional balanced.

When the heart chakra is balanced, our highest self will reside here. Unblocking the heart chakra releases tearful feelings of sadness, the sadness that we have repressed for a lifetime within our being. This brings a sense of relief that is follow by bliss and self-acceptance. Life will appear more joyful and we will appreciate ourselves more, becoming more compassionate not only to ourselves but to others as well.

Throat Chakra

The throat chakra is located over the front and back of the throat area. Its color is blue. The throat chakra's main orientation is with the areas of communication and the expression of creativity via the spoken word, thought and writing. This chakra becomes functional when we commit to expressing our truth to the best of our ability. Our creative desires and aspirations are given birth through the spoken word. This is the home of self-expression and our creative identity. Nothing compares to our ability to be able to communicate truths, wisdom and our personal ideas to others when we communicate from the depth of our inner wisdom. This creates profound internal healing. Through the throat chakra we have the ability to stand up for ourselves and proclaim who we are and our truth.

The use of essential oils is ideal to unblock this chakra center. The throat chakra releases our vocal expressions, giving us the ability to say what we need to say.

Third Eye Chakra

The third eye chakra is located in the center of the brow, just behind the eyes. Its color is purple. The third eye or brow chakra is associated with psychic power, high intuition, inspiration, awareness, and energies of spirit, magnetic forces and light. It also make us aware of the right thinking, about who we are, and it helps us through the difficulties that arise in the world. The brow chakra is the center of divine thought and intuition. Our dreams, visions, intuitive wisdom, intellect and imagination all stem from the third eye chakra. This chakra teaches us to make wise choices, enhances non-verbal communication and helps us express our ideas and thoughts through other creative channels, such telepathy, art, poetry.

When the third eye chakra is fully open, we are able to gain new clarity and understanding about how the world works, and we are easily able to access states of peace, meditation and silence. Our ability to see the world through the eyes of others is also highly enhanced due to our ability to have a heighten sense of consciousness and we part of oneness.

Crown Chakra

The crown chakra is located at the crown of the head, at the center, point upwards. Its color is white. It rules our psyche and our physical and mental well-being. The crown chakra opens our spiritual understanding of the oneness of life. We perceive the world as part of the cosmos and see everyone as perfect piece of the puzzle through the crown chakra. Through it we can make our dreams reality and find personal happiness. A higher power moves our lives in a caring loving way. It gives us an internal and external openness and we understand that everyone is divine, and we love and accept ourselves even more. The crown chakra enables us to see the truth concerning illusory ideals, and to see through pride and vanity.

When the crown chakra is operating fully all boundaries of self disappear and we become ecstatically combined with the whole of existence. We see everything through the eyes of perfect existence and meaning, and with a perfect connection with the inner spirit.

Balance the Chakras

After identifying which chakra may be blocked or unbalanced select the oil or blend of oils according to the suggested chakra aromatherapy oils in Table 1. Use your intuition and your own personal preferences. Please pay attention to any particular allergies or sensitivities to an aroma and select the ideal one for you. Pick your oils and mentally say what they are for. Hold the bottle in your hand and transfer your intent to the oil. Visualize your desires for those oils and close with a simple blessing. Add five drops of chosen oil or blend of oils to 10 mls of carrier oil. Now anoint yourself with your chakra balancing blend on the chakra areas that you feel needs the attention.

Mystical Properties of Some Plants

Not only can essential oils be used to help balance our chakras, many essential oils also have mystical properties. The properties of some of the most common essential oils are presented below.

Basil

Basil is a symbol of fertility and in Italy basil is known as the symbol of love because the leaves resemble hearts. The Basil deva (plant spirit) is a protector of family, and burning basil oil will help to exorcise negativity from the home and bring good luck and happiness to a new home. Basil also has the reputation of being an ideal plant to attract deities and gods. This aromatic plant is worshipped by

Vaishnavite devotees and is used in remedies for various disorders, from the common cold to malaria.

Basil is an adaptogen and has been used to aid meditation and deliver nutrients to the mind that are necessary for the experience of enlivened consciousness. This aromatic plant might be used as aids to elevate the mood and spirit and to calm the mind.

In ayurveda tradition, basil is extensively use for spiritual balancing, use as a food additive, perfume and elixir. Also basil is a powerful tonic and heals the energetic system. It softens the heart chakra, creates inner calmness and promote devotion (bhakti).

Cypress

Essential oils extracted from cypress contain components like alpha pinene, beta pinene, alpha terpinene, bornyl Acetate, camphene, cedrol, cadinene, myrcene, terpinolene and linalool, which acount for its medicinal properties. Cypress is commonly used for blessing, consecration and protection and is commonly use in earth-centered spirituality. Cypress stimulates healing, and helps to ease the anxiety by providing comfort and solace. Cypress wood has been recommended to use in the making the frames for of scrying mirrors that will be used to help the diviner recall past lives.

Cypress wood has long been associated with the everlasting nature of the soul. It been known that spirit boards made from Cypress wood are ideal in ceremonial sessions, rituals and communication with the deceased. In addition, Cypress wood used when spell casting aids in the longevity of the spell.

Cypress essences provide inner strength and quietude, and is useful in times of transition. The cypress tree represents the sacred tree of life, the unchangeable, eternal essence. Some ancient cultures used cypress as a symbol for long life, and eternity. Also cypress is a sign of incorruptibility and remembrance of the purity of the soul. Cypress assists in the rituals regarding sensuality by helping those seeking to transmute the instinctual sex energy into a spiritual energy to experience eternal life. Cypress is an overwhelmingly positive tree and it is also associated with harmony, peace, inspiration, wisdom, cleansing, and psychic defense

Cedar wood

Cedar wood is a purifier, and is beneficial for healing on both the physical and spiritual levels. I (Rose) started to appreciate Cedar trees much more after reading the book, *Anastasia and the Ringing Cedars*, by Vladimir Megre.

These books are based on the ringing cedars which are found in Siberia and can reach heights of forty meters (130 feet) and live to be 550 years old. It is said that these trees sing beautiful songs and they capture the essence of cosmic planetary energies. According to tradition, all the planets pass overhead and reflect cosmic energy down upon the ringing cedars.

Cedars are flexible and receive energy emanating from human consciousness which is reflected back from space. The cedars store this energy and at the right moment give it back to humanity and to every thing living growing on the Earth. Vladimir Megre in <u>Anastasia</u> (p. 6) wrote that, "God created the cedar to store cosmic energy . . . ".

People who are attuned to nature are able to hear the singing of these trees. If we open our hearts we will be able to connect even more with this wonderful tree and receive messages of peace, harmony and healing.

Cedar wood cleanses and purifies the body, skin and the environment from all negativity and stagnation and is a useful oil for overcoming bad habits. Cedar wood enhances clarity of mind and enhances spirituality by helping one to reconnect to their spiritual awareness. The scent is said to enhance psychic powers. Cedar wood harmonizes and stabilizes unbalanced frequencies in our bodies and creates a great shield of protection against other negative, low-vibrational influences. Use Cedar wood to draw Earth energy and for grounding. Cedar wood symbolizes and encourages power, strength and fortitude.

Fennel

Fennel has long been associated with longevity, courage and strength. Fennel wards off negative energies by its purifying properties. Fennel is said to help influence people to trust. It is used in protection charms for both people and property, and in healing and purification rituals. Fennel is additionally said to promote clairvoyance, longevity, and fertility. Metaphysical practitioners use the oil to enhance personal courage and strength. Fennel is recognized as a powerful tool in keeping negative energies at bay, and is often combined with other similar herbs in rites of divination, meditation, and psychic protection.

Frankincense

Frankincense was used by the Egyptians to aid the release of the soul from the body in spiritual ceremonies. This facilitated the connection with Spirit, and raised the level of consciousness. In the process of release, frankincense brought strength and protection. It was often combined in a recipe for anointment with cypress and cedar wood. The essential oil made a wonderful anointing oil for purification and healing, and for connection with the inner self. The use of this combination is not specified, but cypress and cedar wood are both oils of preservation and used for transition into the afterlife. Frankincense was also used in the embalming process in ancient Egypt. Frankincense increases the potency of other oils and is related to sun energy.

Frankincense elevates personal and spiritual love and heightens awareness on all levels by inspiring and awakening the spiritual senses. Frankincense is an oil of transformation that expands consciousness; it is said frankincense accelerates spiritual growth as it promotes the meditative state and opens the crown chakra, causing the energy bodies to drop into alignment and anchor in the physical. A cleanser of the body, aura, psychic planes and environment, frankincense removes all negative influences. Use frankincense oil for; protection, spirituality, love, consecration, blessing, energy, strength, visions, healing, meditation, purification, power and courage.

Geranium

Geranium essential oil has a harmonizing effect on the mind and emotions which makes it wonderful for treating stress. It relaxes the mind and easy the fearful thoughts.

Geranium is use as a protection essence and keeps lower vibrations away, and provides a balancing, uplifting vibration. Geranium has the closest yin/yang balance of all the essential oils and can be used to integrate the differences of male and female energies. Geranium encourages communication, strengthens the throat chakra and enhances the connections to others through the psychic grid. Geranium is also thought to strengthen the etheric body, making it ideal for astral voyages and lucid dreaming. Use geranium oil in rituals invoking love and sensuality, it always attracts romantic feelings and makes us serene and open to receive and give love, similar vibrations than those of rose essences.

Jasmine

Jasmine has a wonderful seductive and sensual aroma. It has been a favorite fragrance oil for many for thousands of years. The name Jasmine comes from the Persian word 'yasmin' which means "a gift from God".

Jasmine is a creeper with white or yellow flowers with an absolutely exquisite scent. It blends well with Rose and geranium, and they carry a fine vibration of delight and love. It is considered a fine and expensive fragrance with delicate, soothing sensations. It is the sacred flower of the Hindu god of love-Kama, and has been used throughout history as a ingredient for love potions or spells to capture or sustain the affection of a loved one. Jasmine is symbolic of the bond of love and passion that is used to unite a bridal couple for eternity. Jasmine also symbolizes the power of the moon over humans, and of the mysteries of the night, Jasmine essential oil is a very soothing, calming and revitalizing oil. This makes it very valuable for mild to severe depression because it soothes the nerves while restoring optimism and energy. As a holistic mystic, I (Rosa) consider the use of jasmine valuable for astral projections and lucid dreaming. The use of jasmine during the night time opens our crown chakra to receive prophetic dreams.

Lavender

The mere mention of lavender brings to mind fields in France, relaxation, and a peaceful day at your favorite spa. Not only does lavender have a pleasing scent, but its healing properties are extensive. The word lavender is already full and vibrant of sacred geometry. You can just visualize lavender flowers or a lavender field to release serotonin and calm feelings and emotions.

Lavender dates as far back as the early Egyptians. The Egyptians wrapped their dead in lavender dipped shrouds. For love, peace and good health, place Lavender flowers in a sachet to be carried on the person. Carrying a sachet containing lavender is also said to attract gentle spirits. Fresh or dried flowers can be rubbed on clothing for romance into one's life. For peaceful sleep, use a few drops of essential oil on the sheets or pillows before bed. For relaxation, purification baths, or aromatherapy purposes, run bathwater over fresh sprigs or place a few drops of oil in the bath. Lavender also provides relaxing properties when taken as a tea. Make a tea from fresh or dried lavender flowers for relaxation, peace, health, and love.

The aroma of lavender is said to stimulate the conscious mind and stabilize both the emotional and etheric planes. It is recommended to use a lavender eye pillow to achieve peaceful dreams and wonderful astral voyages.

Myrrh

Myrrh was used by ancient Egyptians as an offering to Ra, the sun god, they burned the plant and the smoke rose up to the heavens to connect with the gods. They also used it for embalming (it was thought to have antibacterial properties) so it could accompany a soul to the afterlife and because Myrrh is thought to unite heaven and Earth by awakening your awareness of different dimensions. In Kundalini, it is used to strengthen the bond between the crown (heaven) and base (Earth) chakras. It also helps you stay present and not worry about the future. It is often used as an incense.

Myrrh lifts vibrations and increases the potency of other oils. Myrrh has the ability to bring up deep, hidden, or unconscious feelings. Myrrh is purifying to the energetic environment creating very pleasant environments. You can burn myrrh to clean an area of negative energies. Myrrh is an ingredient in healing mixtures and is also used to consecrate, purify and bless objects. Burn myrrh to create sacred spaces, it cleanses the environment and create a sense of inner connection with our own senses promoting pray and meditation.

Orange

Orange is a solar oil that gives us a feeling of warmth and happiness. It also inspires creativity. The orange is a symbol of innocence and fertility and is also a symbol of seduction. Orange is thought to attract abundance and happiness through love and marriage. It is can lift our spirits and help us to feel relaxed and balanced. It is ideal for calming restless children and it sweet aroma bring out sweet memories. Orange harmonizes the body, mind and spirit. Sweet orange essential oil benefits include its antidepressant qualities enabling its users to feel uplifted as well as relaxed. It also boosts the immune system and helps cure colds. Orange awakens creativity, playfulness and enhances the spiritual aspects of life. Orange essential oil can be of great benefit in creating a light and joyful atmosphere, especially in the cold darkness of winter,

Patchouli

Patchouli is a well-known aphrodisiac with magical powers and has been an ingredient in love potions and romantic magic throughout the ages to promote love and sex. Patchouli is also used for meditation practices to ground and center the mind and body.

Patchouli stimulates and balances the yin or feminine aspects and awakens fertility. Usually females use patchouli as a perfume or to increase femininity. Patchouli also promotes physical stamina and increases physical energy and sexual potency. Energetically, patchouli increases attention at the sensory levels and the outer fields, making the person more sensitive to other-worldly experiences, spiritual encounters with mythical creatures and creating an aura of mystery. According to some mystics patchouli also slows down the sense of time perception.

Rose

Rose is the queen of essential oil (and also the most expensive by far) and is also known as the flower of seduction. Rose activates yin or feminine energies and awakens sensuality. It is a healing and balancing oil with a natural affinity with the heart. Rose has the highest frequency of any oil, and raises the frequency of cells bringing harmony and enhanced well-being to the body and balancing personal will. Rose offers psychic protection by raising the energy field frequency. Rose symbolizes real love and attracts love, promotes confidence and is healing to the heart. Giving a single white rose expresses forgiveness. A bouquet of a dozen roses means "true love" because 12 is considered by many religions as a complete cycle. A dozen roses also symbolizes perfection and completeness because of the prominence the number 12 has in natural cycles (12 months in a year) and in religious and mythological traditions (12 apostles, 12 zodiac signs). Nine roses stand for eternal love. Two dozen or three dozen roses express ever deeper feelings of adoration or appreciation. Nine dozen red roses (108 blooms) are a traditional accompaniment to a marriage proposal.

Rosemary

Rosemary was considered a sacred plant in many ancient cultures. In ancient Egypt rosemary was placed in the tomb to remember the dead, used in the bouquets of funeral flowers and even used in the embalming process. Rosemary is believed to strengthen and fortify the memory. People from ancient Greece would place it in their pillow the night to enhance memory during sleep. Use rosemary for cleansing, consecration, peace of mind, release and all kinds of psychic, spiritual and even physical purification. When burned, Rosemary oil emits powerful cleansing and purifying vibrations, and is used to rid a place of negativity. It can be used to cleanses your working space especially prior to performing magic. Rosemary also purifies the human energy fields. Rosemary is an emblem of fidelity for lovers, and can be added to love and lust potions. Rosemary has been used for Remembrance in many ways for centuries, in weddings, funerals, and in daily life as a general memory aid. Use rosemary for any kind of healing rituals.

Sage

Raise your vibrations to slough of the mundane worries that keep your spirit heavy and your thoughts dark with sage. Sage's transformative properties work upon negative energies that are somehow clouding the aura, changing these negative influences to enable them to act for the benefit of the person, place or object whose aura is being cleansed. I personally use sage essential oils to clear my sacred space and home as an alternative to smudging. Sage's scent permeates the environment and creates a barrier of protection-a psychic shield, while neutralizing the existing negativity or misfortune. Sage drives away disturbances and tensions, and lifts the spirits creating an aura of peace by removing dense vibrations from the environment.

Smokeless smudge spray is the pure alternative to burning sage. Whether you need to change the energy or just lighten the air, just one spritz and the wonderful aroma of this spray creates a clean and blessed atmosphere. This quick and easy smudge spray can be use in any cleansing ritual use. Sage enhances the connection to higher self, spirit world, other dimensions and can be used to assist with contacting one's own spiritual guides or animal guides.

Sandalwood

Sandalwood fragrance is woody sweet, and clean. The scent of sandalwood essential oil or sandalwood incense clarifies the mind and helps to awaken intelligence, and is often used as an aid for meditation. It calms the mind, soothes stress and nervous tension, and uplifts the mood. It is said to enliven courage, purpose, strength and happiness. The scent is uplifting, vibrant and good for the magic of divination. It attracts luck, wellbeing and success.

It is thought that sandalwood guides away the distractions of the mind. The sensual joy of the body-the oil is said to predispose the body and mind to sexual ecstasy. Sandalwood has one of the highest vibrations of any oil that resonates with aspects of ourselves, attracting the highest spiritual vibrations, also helps us center our minds in a space of pure serenity and communion with nature. The aromas transport the meditator to a place of bliss. It opens our spiritual centers and aligns the chakras to enhance spiritual awareness, allowing healing energies to flow. Sandalwood enhances receptivity and assists in contact with guardian angels, Devic beings and the higher self. Sandalwood oil placed on the forehead aids in focusing the mind, opens the third eye and facilitates the connection with angelic beings. It also promotes pleasant visions during dream state.

Four

Essential Oil Production and Quality Considerations

The production of essential oils begins with the harvest of the appropriate parts of the desired plants. Some essential oils are derived from flowers, others from leaves, and others from almost the entire plant. To maximize essential oil quality and production the harvest must take place during the correct month and at a certain time of day. Portable distillation units are usually used so that distillation can take place in the field where the plants were grown. This procedure ensures that the essential oils are fresh and also helps maximize production.

The most common methods of essential oil extraction are steam vapor distillation, cold pressing, effleurage, extraction by means of chemical solvents, and carbon dioxide extraction.

Steam Distillation

Steam distillation is the most common method of essential oil extraction and one of the methods which results very high quality oil. The vegetable matter is placed in a distillation basket and the distillation chamber is closed. Steam begins to circulate within the distillation chamber and, when the appropriate temperature is reached, the intercellular cavities in the vegetable matter where the oil is found open. The temperature of the vapor is critical; if the vapor is not hot enough then intercellular cavities don't open and no oil is extracted. On the other hand, if the vapor is too hot then the chemical properties of the essential oil will be altered or the oil will be burned.

The oil evaporates and mixes with the steam vapor when it is released from the intercellular cavities. The oil-laden vapor passes through a cooling tube and enters into a condensation chamber. As the vapor cools it condenses and forms water. Oil, because it is less dense than water, floats on the surface of the water and can be separated and descanted.

The water which remains after the essential oil has been removed is known as *flower water, distillate, or hydrosol*. This water has been "contaminated" by the essential oil and retains some of its properties. Consequently distillate is used in skin-care products and can be preferable for use by persons with very sensitive skin or for new-born babies. Some aromatherapists have started to use hydrosols for their therapeutic value.

Cold Pressing

Cold pressing is used to obtain essential oils from citrus fruits like lemon, mandarin, orange and tangerine. The fruit is passed through a tumbler that is lined with small, sharp knives that penetrate the fruit's thick peel. The fruit is then pressed and juice, pulp and essential oils are squeezed out. The oil, juice and pulp are then separated in a centrifuge.

Effleurage

Some flowers, like jasmine or orange blossom either contain too little essential oil or they are to delicate to undergo steam extraction; heat would destroy the oil before it could be extracted. Effleurage is used in these cases to extract the essential oils from the flowers. The flower pedals are placed on a sheet of vegetable oil or animal fat. These sheets absorb the essential oils from the flowers. Once all of the oil which can be extracted from the flowers has been absorbed the flowers are replaced with new ones. This process continues until the sheets of oil or fat are saturated with essential oil. Alcohol is used to extract the essential oil from the sheets. The essential oils remain after the alcohol evaporates.

Extraction Using Solvents

Extraction by solvents is also used with delicate flowers. This method is less expensive and usually results in the extraction of a greater quantity of essential oil. The vegetable matter is saturated with a chemical solvent. The solvent mixes with the essential oils and the resulting mixture is called a *concrete*. The essential oils are extracted from the concrete by adding alcohol to the mixture. The alcohol and chemical solvent evaporate leaving an *absolute*.

One of the disadvantages of solvent-based extraction is that it is impossible to remove all of the chemical solvent from the absolute. Consequently absolutes are used in the formulation of fragrances and perfumes. However, they should not be therapeutically applied to the skin.

Carbon Dioxide Extraction

Carbon dioxide extraction is one of the more recent technological advances in essential oil extraction. The primary benefit of this method is that it doesn't leave any chemical residues behind. The vegetable material is placed in a pressure vessel and carbon dioxide is injected under pressure. Under pressure the carbon dioxide gas liquefies and works like a chemical solvent, extracting the essential oils from the vegetable matter. When the pressure is released the CO_2 returns to its gaseous state and the essential oils, which are liquid at normal pressure, are released.

The aromas of many essential oils are fresher and more like the aromas of the natural plants when they are extracted using CO_2. In addition, studies have demonstrated that essential oils extracted using this methods are more potent and that they have more therapeutic properties than do oils extracted using other extraction methods.

Essential Oils vs. Synthetic Substitutes

Essential oils come from plants while synthetic substitutes are fabricated in laboratories using petroleum-based products. Aromatherapy requires the use of natural essential oils, not synthetic substitutes. Synthetic substitutes can never bring about the same desired results as those produced when essential oils are used. The reason for this is very simple. An essential oil may contain many chemical compounds. Chemists, when they synthesize a chemical substitute, try to replicate the smell, not the therapeutic properties, of the natural oil. To do this they try to copy a few of the chemical compounds found in the essential oil, those that are primarily responsible for the desired odor. However, the chemical components of the essential oil function synergistically and the synergy is lost when a few, rather than all, of the chemical compounds are copied. You should always verify that you are purchasing pure essential oils for aromatherapy.

Essential Oil Quality

You should pay attention to several factors when you purchase essential oils to ensure that you invest in high quality oils. Some vendors add natural or synthetic products to their oils to alter the appearance, chemical composition or odor of their oils. Other vendors try to improve their profit margins by combining their essential oils with base oil, diluting the essential oil. The practice of adding base oils to essential oils is always acceptable, and is something that you will learn how to do in this course, but the resulting product should be labeled as such. Make sure that the labels of the essential oils which you purchase indicate that the oils are "pure and natural essential oils".

The prices of essential oils are another sign of quality. As always, you get what you pay for. Some companies sell all of their essential oils for the same price. This should be a warning sign to you that the oils are probably chemical synthetics. The prices of pure and natural essential oils are a function of the effort and raw materials required to produce the oils. It takes about 50 pounds of eucalyptus, 150 pounds of lavender, 500 pounds of rosemary, 1,000 pounds of jasmine and over 2,000 pounds of rose to make a single pound of essential oil! The price of each essential oil is directly related to the amount of plant material needed for distillation. The table below shows the current year (2011) retail prices for 0.5 ml of common essential oils.

As you can see in Table 1, the prices of essential oils vary substantially. If the label on an essential oil bottle doesn't say that the bottle contains "essential oil" or "pure essential oil" or "natural essential oil" chances are good that it isn't an essential oil. A bottle of "perfumed oil" is not essential oil; most likely it is a base oils that has been "perfumed" with a chemical substitute. If the label says that the oil is "identical" to the natural oil then you have just been warned that the contents are a chemical synthetic that has been formulated to imitate the aroma and chemical composition of an essential oil. These oils can not be identical because they lack the vital energy or life force derived from living plant matter. In addition, the chemical synthetics, as noted above, replicate the few chemical components responsible for odor and lack the hundreds of other components which account for the therapeutic value of essential oils. Please remember that *only true essential oils come from plants and only from plants.*

Table 1
Essential Oil Prices[1]

Essential Oil	Retail Price (.5 fl oz)[2]
Bergamot	$13.59
Chamomile, Roman	19.49
Clary Sage	13.39
Eucalyptus	5.99
Frankincense	28.39
Geranium	17.51
Lavender, Harvest	10.19
Lemon	5.49
Myrrh	23.19
Patchouli, Dark	19.70
Peppermint	8.99
Rose, Absolute	59.39
Rose, Otto	101.72
Rosemary	6.42
Tea Tree	8.59
Thyme, Red	16.94
Ylang Ylang	14.99

Finally, "impregnated" oils are not pure essential oils. Impregnated oils are base oils in which vegetable matter has been soaked or cooked. The base oil become impregnated with some of the components of the essential oil and may carry some of the therapeutic properties and aroma on an essential oil. The most common impregnated oils are chamomile, aloe, arnica, marigold, comfrey, mullein, and hypericum.

---

[1]   Prices from Aura Cacia accessed at www.auracacia.com on 19 May 2017.

[2]   Except for Rose and Chamomile which are 0.125 fl oz.

Care of Essential Oils

Essential oils are sensitive to light, heat and air. The properties of the oils change rapidly with exposure to any of these three factors. Consequently it is very important that you store you essential oils in a dark, cool and dry location in your home or office. Do not store your oils in the bathroom because humidity will affect the oils. Essential oils should always be stored in amber-colored jars and you should leave the jars open just long enough to obtain the drops of oil that you may need. This will ensure that the volatile oils do not evaporate and that contact with the air does not change their chemical composition. Your jars of essential oil should never be opened for more than a few seconds.

Five

Introduction to Human Physiology

Aromatherapy functions on at least two levels in the human body: the physical level and the emotional level. Although it is difficult to measure, some feel that aromatherapy also affects our spiritual level. Although you can't scientifically measure the spiritual effects of aromtherapy you may be able to feel them in your life.

Aromatherapy achieves its physical effects through absorption through the skin and through the lungs. The following sections explain how aromatherapy works on a physical level.

Absorption through the Skin

We often forget that our skin is an organ and that the application of substances to the skin can affect our bodies. Many think of the skin only as a covering that keeps foreign matter out of our bodies and keeps our organs and muscles inside. René Gattefossé demonstrated that the skin is able to absorb oils when their molecular structure is sufficiently small. Even so, it is difficult for some to believe that the body is able to absorb essential oils. Remember however that one of the most common medical treatments for the symptoms of menopause is the administration of estrogen by means of small patches that are applied to the skin, or in other words, the application of estrogen by absorption through the skin. Figure 1 below shows the structure of your skin. You can see the capillaries in the dermis in the diagram.

Figure 1
The Skin

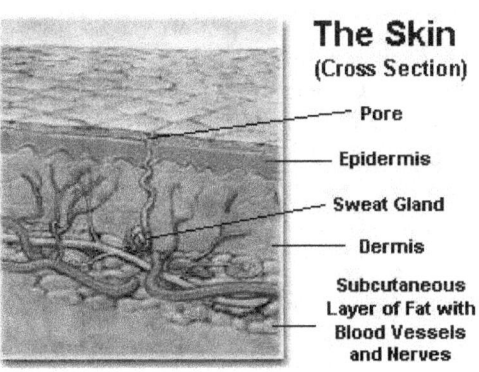

The Skin
(Cross Section)

- Pore
- Epidermis
- Sweat Gland
- Dermis
- Subcutaneous Layer of Fat with Blood Vessels and Nerves

Essential oils have a very small molecular structure. The oil molecules enter the body through the follicle capillaries that contain an oily liquid called sebum. Essential oils have an affinity for sebum because they are both oil-based. The essential oils are then enter the lymphatic system and are transported to other parts of the body. This entire process takes place in just a few minutes.

The lymphatic system is an often-overlooked part of the circulatory system. As blood passes through the capillaries, some of the fluid diffuses into the surrounding tissues. One function of the lymphatic system is to collect and recycle this fluid (called lymph). Lymph passes from capillaries to lymph vessels and flows through lymph nodes that are located along the course of these vessels. Cells of the lymph nodes *phagocytize,* or ingest, impurities such as bacteria, old red blood cells, and toxic and cellular waste. Finally, lymph flows into the thoracic duct, a large vessel that runs parallel to the spinal column, or into the right lymphatic duct, both of which transport the lymph back into veins of the shoulder areas where iy mixes with blood and is returned to the heart. Thus essential oils which enter the body through the skin finally enter into the blood flow. All lymph vessels contain one-way valves, like the veins, to prevent backflow.

The tissues of the lymphatic system include the spleen. The spleen serves as a reservoir for blood, releasing additional blood into the circulatory system as needed. It is also involved with destruction of old cells and other substances by *phagocytosis.* The lymphatic system is also responsible for collecting nutrients that the digestive system has extracted from our foods, and is a very important part of the immune system.

Figure 2 below shows the structure of the lymphatic system.Essential oil molecules affect the body in much the same way as do herbal medicines. Different essential oils have affinities for different systems and organs. For example juniper and cypress have an affinity for the kidneys. Geranium and basil influence hormone levels by effecting the suprarenal cortex and bergamot and geranium have a "normalizing" effect on both the mind and the body.

Figure 2
The Lymphatic System

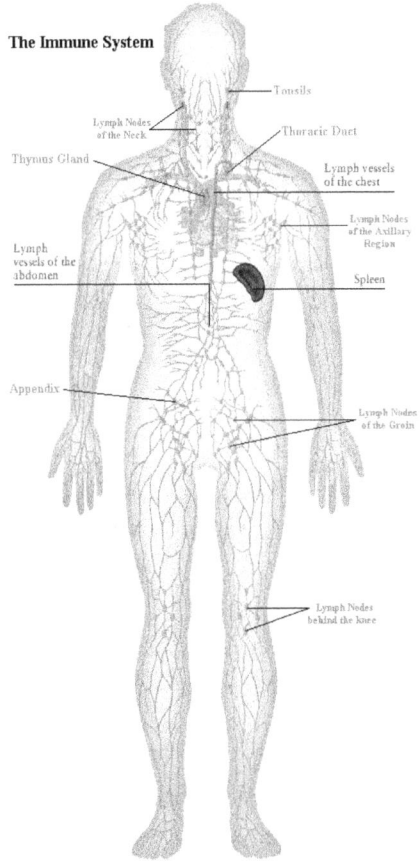

The Immune System

Tonsils

Lymph Nodes of the Neck

Thoracic Duct

Thymus Gland

Lymph vessels of the chest

Lymph Nodes of the Axillary Region

Lymph vessels of the abdomen

Spleen

Appendix

Lymph Nodes of the Groin

Lymph Nodes behind the knee

Figure 3 summarizes the flow of essential oils through the body when they are applied to the skin. It takes twenty to ninety minutes for essential oils to be entirely absorbed into the body, and another three to six hours for the oils to be excreted from a healthy body. It may take up to three times as long for the essential oils to be excreted from an unhealthy body. As shown in the diagram below, the process of oil absorption through the skin is complex and affects many of the subsystems of your body. Figure 4 below depicts the flow of essential oils when they are administered through inhalation.

Figure 3
Essential Oil Flow -- Skin Application

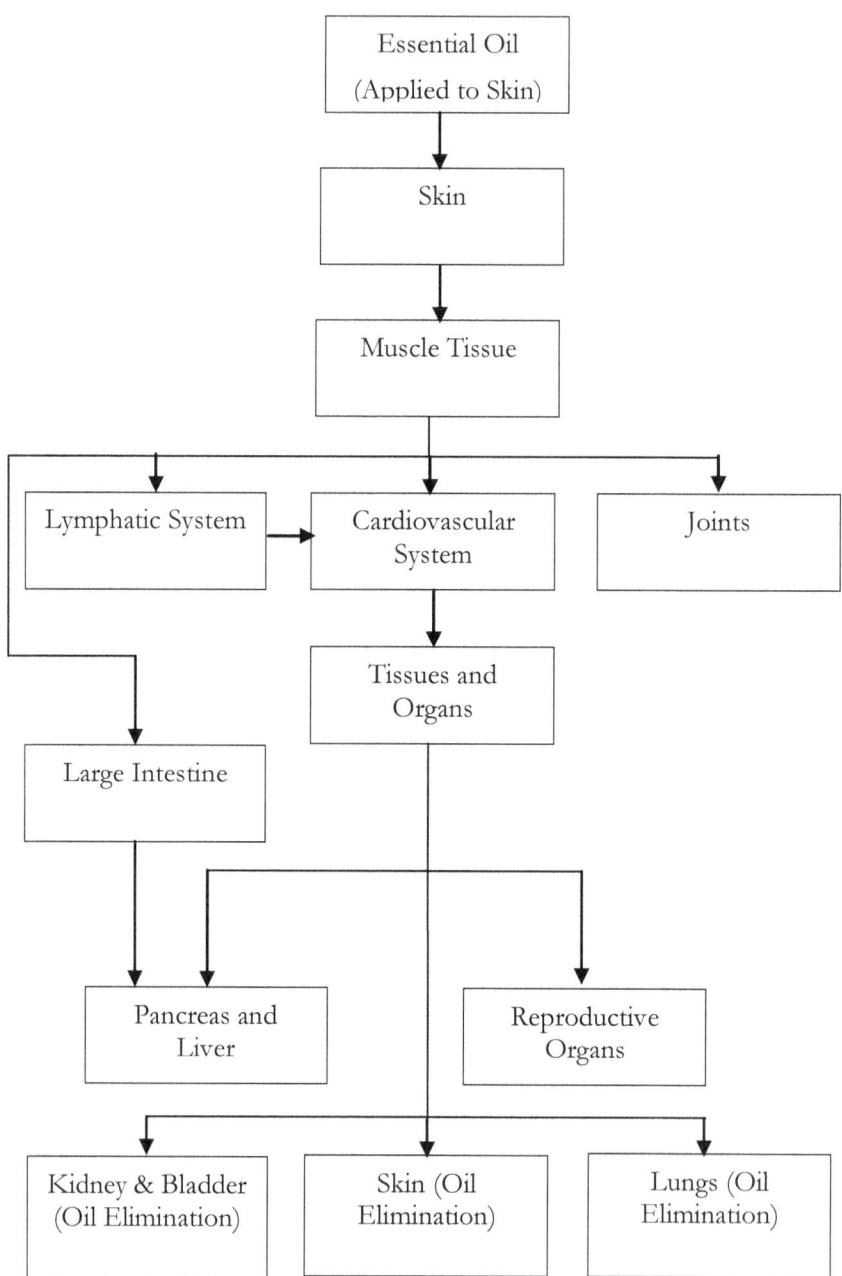

Absorption through the Lungs

Another way that the molecules of aromatic oils enter our bodies is through our lungs. The molecules pass through the air sacks in the lungs and enter the capillary veins and from there into the veins that circulate the oxygen rich blood throughout the body. The inhalations of some substances, like chemical solvents or cocaine have a damaging effect on the body and effects the mind. The inhalation of other substances through respiratory therapy in a hospital or aromatherapy can improve a person's physical and mental health. Figure 4 shows the heart and lungs. The pulmonary veins pick up oxygen and also the essential oil molecules in the lungs. Both are then circulated together throughout the body.

Figure 4
Heart and Lungs

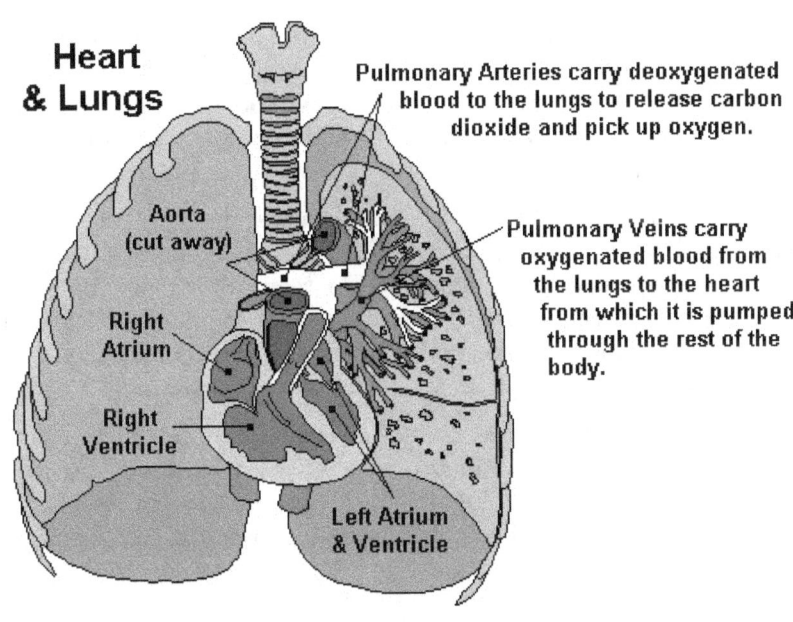

The scientists John Steele and Maxwell Cade have investigated the effects of essential oil inhalation on the mind. In their research they have connected subjects to EEG machines to measure the body's response to various essential oils. Essential oils like rosemary, basil and peppermint, which have traditionally been used to stimulate thought processes, produced an increase in beta waves, the brain waves which indicate an alert mental state. The scientists measured an increase in alpha, theta and delta wave in the minds of the subjects who inhaled essential oils of rose and azar, which have traditionally been used as anti-depressives. Alpha, theta and delta waves indicate a restful state, one that approximates the state of a mind in meditation.

Steve Van Toller and George Dodd[3] at the University of Warwick in England have undertaken a series of studies on the effects of aromas on emotions. They discovered that the skin responds to aromas, even when subjects report that they are not able to detect the aroma. Many people, for example, are not able to detect pheromones even though in all other respects their sense of smell is normal. In one experiment subjects were connected to an EEG machine which registered skin and brain responses. The equipment registered significant skin responses to pheromones even when the volunteers reported that they could not detect an aroma.

In other studies they discovered that people are able to block the central nervous system effects of aromas that they don't like. This finding is important for aromatherapists. We should not force clients to accept aromas that they don't like. In addition, it is a good idea to let the clients help select the aromas which we will use in a treatment.

A common criticism of aromatherapy is that our sense of smell tires rapidly. The olfactory cells in the nose stop functioning when they become overloaded or saturated. Consequently, some argue that aromatherapy effects are short lived. However Marguerite Maury[4] has demonstrated that the emotional and physical effects of essential oils last after the sense of smell ceased to detect the aromas.

The chain of effects of essential oils when they are inhaled is shown on the next page in Figure 5. Note that inhaled oils also affect the cardiovascular system (Figure 4). You will recall that essential oils which enter the lungs absorbed into the blood stream and distributed throughout the body.

---

[3]   Dodd, G. and S. Van Toller, *Perfumery*, Chapman and Hall, 1988.

[4]   Maury, M. *The Secret of Life and Youth*, C. W. Daniel, 1989.

Figure 5
Essential Oil Flow -- Inhalation

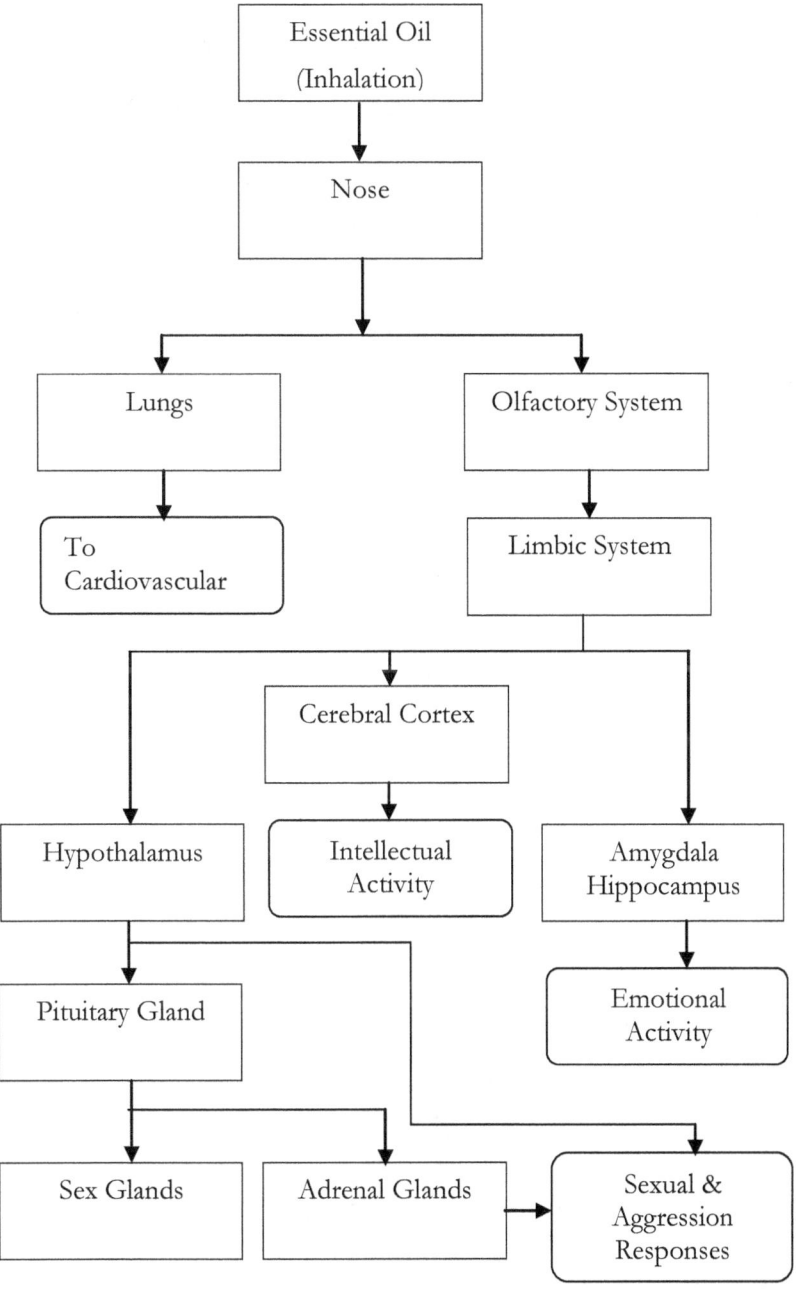

Recall that the cardiovascular that the cardiovascular system supplies blood to all organs so, to some degree, the organs in this figure are also influenced by essential oils applied to the skin.

Body Systems

A system is a set of interrelated parts which work together to achieve some goal. The goal of your body is to keep you alive and healthy. To do that your body relies on eight major subsystems. Table 2 summarizes the functions and common concerns for each of the major subsystems. Not all of the health concerns listed in Table 2 are normally treated by aromatherapy. Through continued study and practice you will discover which conditions are most susceptible to aromatherapy and when it is appropriate to suggest an alternative health treatment (herbs, homeopathic remedies, or Bach flower remedies for example) to your clients.

Table 2
Body Subsystems

Subsystem	Function	Common Concerns
Digestive	The Grocery Store Breaks food down for fuel and makes it available to the whole body	Indigestion Heartburn Insufficient enzymes Stomach ulcers Stomach cramps
Intestinal	Waste Disposal Plant Absorbs waste products from the body and excretes those products with indigestible food fiber	Constipation/diarrhea Hemorrhoids Diverticulitis Colitis Crohn's disease Irritable bowel syndrome
Circulatory	The Center of Life Transports food, oxygen and water to every subsystem in the body	Cholesterol/triglycerid buildup Hypertension Arterial plaque Stress Poor circulation Heart disease
Nervous	Communication Network Provides the communication link between our body and the external world	Headaches Insomnia Nervous disorders Depression Memory loss

Immune	Security System--	Viral/bacterial attack
	Recognizes viruses, bacteria and other foreign bodies and	Fatigue
		Stress
		Cancer
Respiratory	Oxygen Supplier	Asthma
	Supplies oxygen which is necessary to produce energy	Hay fever
		Coughs
		Bronchitis
Urinary	Water-Treatment Plant	Bladder/kidney infection
	Passes the water within our body through a filtration process to maintain a clean supply of fluids that the body can use	Kidney stones
		Incontinence
		Cystitis
		Pain and irritation
Glandular	Body's Thermostat	Hormone imbalance
	A communication network that regulates basic drives and emotions, promotes growth and sexual identity, assists in the repair of broken tissues and helps generate energy	Emotional stress
		Reproductive problems
		Hyper/Hypo sugar levels
Structural	The Body's Framework	Arthritis
	Houses our body's other subsystems and helps our body withstand outside stress and strain	Osteoporosis
		Muscle cramps
		Poor posture

Essential oils enter our bodies through the respiratory system (the lungs) and the structural system (the skin). The essential oils are then distributed throughout our bodies by the circulatory system (blood flow) and the immune system (lymphatic flow). However, remember that the essential oils affect more than the systems involved in transport.

Six

Essential oils

In this chapter you will discover the uses and properties of basic essential oils as well as extraction methods, chemical composition, and common uses of an initial repertoire of essential oils. In addition, in this chapter, we review the chemical components of essential oils and some of their effects.

Oil Chemistry

The fundamentals of chemicals in essential oils can be divided into the following functional groups.

1. Terpene

Terpenes are present in most essential oils; they are unsaturated hydrocarbons that are partly responsible for the scent that a plant produces, and can vary from season to season depending on the concentration.

Monoterpenes can stress the kidneys (Juniper). They also function as decongestants of mucous glands. Examples of essential oils that contain monoterpenes include juniper, pine, and sweet orange.

Sesquiterpenes provide essential oils with anti-inflammatory and analgesic properties which are useful in treating muscular aches and pain. An example of an essential oil that contains sesquiterpenes is German chamomile.

2. OLS

Alcohols (Monoterpenols) contain 10 carbon units. These chemicals have solvent actions. That means that they are liquids that are able to dissolve substances to form solutions. Monoterpenols tend to provide an energizing effect as well as having anti-viral, antiseptic and anti-bacterial properties. Essential oils with a high proportion of alcohols are considered to have a low toxicity level and are relatively safe for general use. They are also anti infectious, vasoconstrictors (shrinks veins), and (especially menthol) cause a cold sensation on skin. These chemicals help regulate and boost the immune system. They are good for long term use. Essential oil that contain alcohols include rosewood and tea tree (95% monoterpenes), palma rosa, sweet marjoram, eucalyptus, and lavender.

Sesquiterpenols, another alcohol, contain 15 carbon units. These chemicals have estrogen like properties and help blood flow. Consequently they should not be used by pregnant women. Essential oils that contain sesquiterpenols include patchouli, neroli, cedarwood, and cypress.

Phenols are weak acids that have disinfectant and anti-bacterial as well as stimulating properties. They help to cleanse wounds and treat inflammations. They are also useful as painkillers. Thyme is an example of an essential oil with these attributes. Oils containing these chemicals can be irritating, so they should only be used in low dosages and should never be used neat (full strength). It is a good idea to avoid essential oils with Phenols as they will burn mucus membranes when you smell them.

3. Hydes

Aldehydes are used in the preparation of solvents, and are often responsible for the scent of a plant. They seem to be the main constituents of Lemon, Lemongrass and Melissa. They are skin irritants (if used neat), calming (via olfactory system), anti-infectious, and anti-inflammatory. Examples of essential oils that contain aldehydes include citriadora, eucalyptus, lemon, lemon balm, lemon verbena, and lemongrass.

4. Tones

Ketones resemble aldehydes, but are less reactive, providing a solvent action. They help determine the main characteristics of the essential oil in which they occur. Ketones assist in balancing the flow of mucus. Most aromatherapists feel that oils containing a fair amount of ketones, such as Hyssop and Sage, can be hazardous and should be used with care. Some oils contain the ketone cineole which can, depending upon the concentration, cause significant burning to mucous membranes if accidentally ingested.

Ketones are hepatoxic (they can be toxic to the liver), convulsive in high dosages, and mucolytic (mucous dissolving). Consequently they are often used to treat respiratory problems. Examples of essential oils that contain ketones include camphor, eucalyptus, peppermint, and spearmint.

Diketones have wound and scar healing properties and reduce bruising. Everlasting is an example of an essential oil that contains diketones.

5. Esters

Esters have anti-spasmodic (depending on the underlying parent acid and alcohol combination) central nervous system sedative, and anti-inflammatory properties. Linalyl acetate, a naturally occurring ester, is a biochemical union of the alcohol linalool and acetic acid. It is found in essential oils of lavender, lavendin, lemon, sage, bergamont, jasmin, ylang ylang, cananga, clary sage and neroli. Other examples of essential oils that contain esters include Roman chamomile, sweet marjoram, geranium, and angelica.

Some of these oils are very calming (chamomile, lavender and angelica) for nervous exertion. In large doses they can be stupefying, others are stimulating (clove, tarragon, fennel).

6. Oxides

Oxides are exocrine gland stimulants, and stimulate the mucous glands of respiratory and digestive tract. They are also used for treating dry skin. Examples of oils high in oxides include eucalyptus radiata, and cardomon.

7. Acids

Acids are known to speed up chemical reactions and usually have antiseptic and diuretic properties. They can help to lower fevers.

Common Properties

Most essential oils share the following properties. Properties specific to individual essential oils are discussed in the oil profile section that follows.

- ✓ Anti-bacterial, anti-microbic, anti-virus (the best known is tea tree)
- ✓ Detoxify - gets rid of poisons from our blood stream. Urine is usually yellow; it is a sign of toxins being discarded as it gets darker.
- ✓ Oxygenate - as oxygen is added it has the effect of pumping up the tissues.
- ✓ Temporarily helps rid tissues of excess fluid.
- ✓ Easily absorbed by the skin because they are lipo solvents - they dissolve in fats. They dissolve in the fatty part of the skin to quickly penetrate different layers before entering the bloodstream
- ✓ Has the power of healing rapidly.
- ✓ Help balance the nervous system.
- ✓ Inflammable, and so can ignite.
- ✓ Odoriferant - smelly.
- ✓ Penetrate through the skin.

- ✓ Promote new cell growth and sheds dead skin cells.
- ✓ Improve circulation by regulating the action of capillaries.
- ✓ Regulate and balances body functions (Bergamot, Clary Sage, Lavender, Geranium).
- ✓ Rehydrate over 3-6 hours.
- ✓ Restore vitality to tissues.
- ✓ Soluble in pure alcohol (ethanol), vegetable oils and, to a lesser extent, in water.
- ✓ Volatile - when exposed to air they evaporate quickly.
- ✓ Watery and do not leave an oily mark on paper.

Essential Oil Profiles

The essential oil profiles for a basic repertoire of essential oils are provided below. As a beginning aromatherapist you should be very familiar with the actions and uses of these essential oils:

- Bergamot
- Chamomile (Roman)
- Clary Sage
- Eucalyptus
- Geranium
- Lavender
- Lemon
- Orange
- Patchouli
- Peppermint
- Rose
- Rosemary
- Sandalwood
- Tea Tree
- Ylang Ylang

In the pages below the aromatherapy class (general use), aroma type and perfume note are provided. The profiles also give a description of the essential oil, its common uses, and precautionary notes about the use of the essential oil when appropriate.

BERGAMOT

CITRUS AURANTIUM VAR. BERGAMIA

(Family, Rutaceae)

Aromatherapy Class -- Balancing, Calming

Aroma Type -- Citrus

Perfume Note -- Top

Description -- Common to Northern Africa and Italy, the bergamot tree, a lemon-orange hybrid, grows about fifteen feet tall and is covered with green leaves and small white flowers. It bears a pear-shaped fruit which is a little smaller than an orange. Bergamot oil is derived from the fruit rind of the bergamot tree. The oil, which is often combined with lavender or geranium, smells like a mixture of lemon and orange flowers. You may recognize the scent if you are a tea drinker, it gives Earl Grey tea its distinctive aroma and flavor.

Bergamot blends well with chamomile, coriander, cypress, geranium, juniper, lavender, lemon, neroli, and ylang ylang.

Common Uses -- Bergamot is used to treat gastric or digestive problems. It increases appetite and reduces flatulence and because it has antispasmodic actions it can be used to relieve colic. It also has anti-parasitic properties and can be used as an effective vermifuge.

Bergamot has antiseptic properties and has been used effectively to treat urinary and skin infections such as acne (use in sits baths for urinary infection and in lotions or creams to treat skin conditions).

Bergamot can be used as a sedative for anxiety and to relieve melancholia and as an antidepressant.

It has been traditionally as an antiseptic, deodorant, perfume, soothing agent, skin conditioner

Skin Type: oily, blemished, normal to combination

Main Constituents -- Linalyl acetate (an ester), linalol, sequiterpenes, terpenes, furocoumarins

Extraction Method -- Expressing (hand press)

Safety Information -- Direct application may result in skin irritation or increased photosensitivity.

CHAMOMILE, ROMAN
ANTHEMIS NOBILIS OR *CHAMAEMELUM NOBILE*
(Family, Asteraceae [Compositae])

Aromatherapy Class -- Calming

Aroma Type -- Fruity

Perfume Note -- Middle

Description -- Three different varieties of chamomiles are grown for their essential oils, Roman Chamomile, German Chamomile and Mixed Chamomile. Roman Chamomile, of the three, has the most therapeutic properties. This plant is native to Europe and is grown in Belgium, Bulgaria, England, France, Hungary and Italy. The perennial plant grows to a height of 22 to 30 cm and is covered with small white flowers with yellow centers. The yellowish essential oil is produced from the flowers and leaves of the plant.

Roman Chamomile blends well with galbanum, eucalyptus, and rosemary.

Common Uses -- Chamomile is a wonderful generalist which has traditionally be used as an antispasmodic and relaxant; more recently it has been recognized as an analgesic. It has anti-inflammatory, anti-bacterial and hydrating properties. Consequently it is used to treat a number of skin disorders including acne, boils, burns, dermatitis and rashes. Because it is a sebum solvent it can also be used to relieve pore congestion. It is an effective remedy for gingivitis and as an ophthalmic treatment for conjunctivitis because of its anti-infectious properties

Chamomile's antispasmodic, anticonvulsive and antipyretic properties make it useful in treating cramps and fevers. It is also used for digestive problems including digestive sluggishness, colic, nausea, dyspepsia and ulcers because it is a stomachic and apéritif. Chamomile tea is used frequently in South America after meals to aid digestion and also before bed as a relaxant. It can also be used as a hepatic stimulant in cases of jaundice and biliousness.

The nervine and analgesic properties of Chamomile provide relief from pain and discomfort from gout, migraine, neuralgia, rheumatism, toothache and earache.

The psychological effects of Chamomile are similar to its physiological calming effects[5]. Chamomile is a mild sedative and can be used in cases of anger, anxiety, insomnia, or hysteria. It also has antidepressant properties and can be used to combat nightmares and moodiness. Chamomile is especially safe for children because of its very low toxicity.

Stress causes chemical changes in the body. For example the level of adrenocorticotropic hormone (ACTH) in the blood stream increases when individuals are under stress. Research in Japan shows that inhaling the scent of chamomile oil decreases the plasma levels of ACTH in laboratory rats subjected to stress-inducing restrictions.

Skin Type -- Sensitive

Main Constituents -- Esters, pinene, fanesol, nerolidol, chamazulene, pinocarvone, cineol.

Extraction Method -- Steam distillation. Chamomile's important azulene constituent is formed during distillation.

---

[5]   Yamada, K. et al. "Effect of inhalation of chamomile oil vapor on plasma ACTH level in ovariectomized-rat under restriction stress." *Biological & Pharmaceutical Bulletin*; 1996, 19: 1244-1246.

CLARY SAGE

SALVIA SCLAREA

(Family, Lamiaceae [Labiatae])

Aromatherapy Class -- Balancing, calming, toning

Aroma Type -- Herbaceous

Perfume Note -- Top/middle

Description -- Clary Sage, a biennial, displays its robust pale blue, purple and pink flowers from May to September growing to a three to five feet tall. It was grown originally in the South of France, Italy and Syria and flourishes today in England, Central Europe, Russia, the Morocco and the United States. Its clear or pale yellow-green essential oil is extracted from the flowers and its heart-shaped leaves. The oil has a sweet and fresh aroma with herbal, nut and balsamic matices.

The plant has traditionally been used to flavor German muscatel wine, English beer and Italian vermouth; and as a perfume fixative. Herbologists have traditionally used clary sage to treat digestive disorders, kidney and respiratory infections and sore throat. Note that clary sage (*salvia sclarea*) is not the same as common sage (*salvia officinalis*). The later is toxic and should not be used in aromatherapy.

Clary Sage blends well with Cedarwood, Labdanum, citrus oils, and Lavender Lavandin.

Common Uses -- The term *sclarea* in the Latin name of the plant comes from the root *clarus* which means to clarify or clean. In the Middle Ages the plant was known as eye-bright and was famous as an eye wash.

It has traditionally been used as a skin conditioner, astringent, soothing agent, aphrodisiac, and muscle relaxant. Clary Sage is used to treat a variety of conditions from insomnia and hyperactivity in children, to PMS symptoms and menopause, to feelings of hysteria, panic and paranoia. The chemical makeup of clary sage is similar to that of female hormones (this is due to its sclareol content) and thus it is used to treat female conditions and life changes such as menopause and to stimulate irregular or late menstrual cycles.

The linalyl acetate (an ester) in Clary Sage is responsible for it antispasmodic and sedative properties. This explains its use as an effective antispasmodic and anticonvulsant. It is useful in treating stomach problems like dyspepsia (indigestion) and flatulence, and also headaches, vertigo and sore throats.

The diterpene scalareol and sesquiterpene carypohyllene (terpenoids) found in Clary Sage make it effect in combating the *Staphylococcus aureus, Candida albicans,* and *Proteus mirabilis* bacteria and yeasts.[6]

Skin Type -- Normal to combination

Main Constituents -- Linalyl acetate, linalol, pionene, myrcene, sclareol, phellandrene, and caryophyllene.

Extraction Method -- Steam distillation

Safety Information -- Do not use during pregnancy. Do not drink alcohol or drive when after using Clary Sage. The use of Clary Sage in confined spaces may cause headaches. Overuse may cause an increase in blood pressure and dizziness.

---

[6] Ulubelen, A. et al. "Terpenoids from Salvia sclarea." *Phytochemistry*, 1994, 36(4): 971-974.

EUCALYPTUS

EUCALYPTUS GLOBULUS

(Family, Myrtaceae)

Aromatherapy Class -- Toning, stimulating

Aroma Type -- Camphoraceous

Perfume Note -- Top

Description -- The Eucalyptus tree is native to Australia where more than 75% of the trees are Eucalyptus trees. Aborigines and the first colonists planted them to drain swamps and combat misquotes as well as for their hard wood. Today it is found in areas with climates that are similar that that of the Mediterranean area such as California, Egypt, Hawaii, India, Latin America, Portugal, South Africa, Spain, and Tahiti. The tree can grow to a height of over 450 feet and is covered with dark green leaves. Seed capsules cover the branches of the trees giving the tree its name; *eukalyptos* in Greek means "covered".

There are several hundred varieties of Eucalyptus tree but the *Eucalyptus Globulus* is the most common source of the essential oil used in aromatherapy. You may also find essential oils of *Eucalyptus australiana, Eucalyptusbakeri, Eucalyptus citriodora, Eucalyptus dives, Eucalyptus polybrachtea, Eucalyptus radiata* and *Eucalyptus smithii.* The aroma of the *Eucalyptus Globulus* tree is stimulating, refreshing, penetrating and a little medicinal (camphorous). The aroma of the *Eucalyptus citriodora* tree is similar to the essential oils of citrius trees while the aroma of the *Eucalyptus dives* tree is similar to that of mint.

The essential oil of the *Eucalyptus Globulus* is one of the most versatile or universal oils.

Eucalyptus blends well with coriander, juniper berry, lavender, lemon, lemongrass and thyme.

Common Uses -- Eucalyptus oil has traditionally been used as a deodorant, antiseptic, soothing agent, skin conditioner and insect repellent. The oil is an effective remedy for all types of respiratory ills (colds, cough, sore throat, and sinus problems). It can be used as an inhalant, chest rub, massage oil, sauna, baths and compresses. In the 1940s and 1950s Eucalyptus was the active ingredient in cold and cough medicines because of its strong antibacterial, expectorant and cough suppressing action.

Eucalyptus oil can be used in an atomizer, diffuser or vaporizer to both deodorize (it has a pleasing lemon scent) and as a disinfectant to inhibit contagion. It is also an effective germicidal, anti-parasitic and insect repellent. As an antibacterial it is also useful in treating urinary tract infections, although when used in excess it can tax the kidneys. It can also be used alone or with Bergamot as to reduce the pain and speed the healing of herpes and chicken pox.

Research conducted in India shows that eucalyptus oil is an effective bactericide against *Escherichia coli (E. coli)* strain SP-11. Later studies indicated that it is also an effective antibacterial and antifungal against at least 22 Gram-positive and Gram-negative bacteria and 11 yeast-like and filamentous fungi in vitro including *Cryptococcus neoformans* an AIDS-related opportunistic fungus.[7]

Used in conjunction with Geranium and Juniper, Eucalyptus can be used to regulate blood sugar levels. It also has very effective analgesic properties and can be used to treat migraine headaches, arthritis, rheumatism and muscle pain.

Eucalyptus is an emotional stabilizer and can be used to restore emotional equilibrium, improve concentration and to increase intellectual capacity. *Eucalyptus citriodora* has a sedative effect.

A study conducted at Germany's Neurological Clinic at the University of Kiel demonstrated that the topical application of eucalyptus and peppermint oil to large areas of the forehead and temples produced a muscle-relaxing and mentally relaxing effect. A subsequent study demonstrated that these two oils resulted in a significant temporal muscle-relaxing effect on individuals with experimentally-induced headache pain.[8] This indicates that both oils may be effective in reducing headache pain.

---

[7]   Pattnaik, S. et al. "Effect of essentail oils on the viability and morphology of *Escherichia coli.*" *Microbios*; 1995, 84(340): 195-199. Pattnaik, S. et al.
"Antibacterial and antifunglal activity of ten essential oils in vitro." *Microbios*; 1996, 86(349): 237-246. Viollon, c. and J. P. Chaumont. "Antifungal properties of essential oils and their main components upon *Cryptococcus neoformans.*" *Mycopathologia*; 1994, 128(3): 151-153.

[8]   Gobel, H., et al. "Effect of peppermint and eucalyptus oil preparations on neurphysiological and experimetnal algesimetric headach parameters." *Cephalagia*;

Skin Type -- Blemished

Main Constituents -- Cineole (ecualypto), pinene, limonene, cymene, phellandrene, terpinene, and aromadendrene.

Extraction Method -- Steam distillation

Safety Information -- Eucalyptus can irritate sensitive skin. Eucalyptus oil, like all essential oils, should be kept out of the reach of children. A lethal oral dose of Eucalyptus essential oil for a three year-old child is 5 ml.

1994, 14(3): 228-234. ___. "Essential plant oils and headache mechanisms." *Phytomedicine*; 2(2): 93-102.

This page intentionally blank

GERANIUM
PELARGONIUM GRAVEOLENS
(Family, Geraniaceae)

Aromatherapy Class -- Balancing, soothing

Aroma Type -- Floral

Perfume Note -- Middle to top

Description -- The Geranium flower is native to Southern Africa. While there are over 700 varieties only a few (*pelargonium graveolens, pelargonium odorantissimum,* and *pelargonium radula* are used in essential oil production. Today China, Egypt and islands in the Southwest Indian Ocean are the main producers of this essential oil. The essential oil is a pale yellow-green with a fresh, sweet scent which may be reminiscent of roses or mint.

Geranium combines well with cedarwood, citronella, clary sage, grapefruit, jasmine, lavender, lime, neroli, orange, petitgrain, rose, rosemary and sandalwood.

Common Uses -- Like Eucalyptus, Geranium is one of the aromatherapy universals. It has traditionally been used as a skin refresher and astringent. However, it is an effective diuretic, antiseptic and astringent. It is useful in the treatment of urinary tract infections and for regulating blood sugar levels (anti-diabetic properties). As an anti-microbial, Geranium can be used as a mouthwash or gargle for sore throats and other oral infections.

Research conducted in India shows that geranium oil is an effective antibacterial and antifungal against at least 22 Gram-positive and Gram-negative bacteria and 11 yeast-like and filamentous fungi in vitro.[9]

Geranium affects to adrenal cortex and consequently, nervousness and depression and regulates hormone secretion. It also works as a psychological stimulant that balances and stabilizes.

---

[9] Pattnaik, S. et al. "Antibacterial and antifunglal activity of ten essential oils in vitro." *Microbios*; 1996, 86(349): 237-246.

However, a few individuals find that Geranium is a sedative. This is due to the aldehyde citronellal (which is also found in lemon and rose oils).

Skin Type -- oily, dry

Main Constituents -- Geraniol, borneol, aldehyde citronellal citronellol (a monoterpene alcohol), linalol, termineol, limonene, phellandrene and pinene.

Extraction Method -- Steam distillation of the entire plant

Safety Information -- Geranium should be avoided or used with caution with patients with hypoglycimia or hyperinsulinemia because it quickly lowers blood sugar levels.

LAVENDER

LAVANDULA ANGUSTIFOLIA

(Family, Lamiaceae [Labiatae])

Aromatherapy Class -- Calming, balancing, soothing

Aroma Type -- Herbaceous

Perfume Note -- Middle to top

Description -- Lavender is a perennial bush with blue-violet or purple flowers which grows from 90 to 120 cm tall. The essential oil ranges from clear to pale blue to yellow-green. Its aroma has been described as sweet, floral, herbal, woodsy and balsamic. Although there are more than 30 species of Lavender only four are used frequently in aromatherapy: *Lavandual officinalis, Lavandula angustifolia, Lavandula vera* and *lavandula stoechas*.

Lavender blends well with bergamot, clary sage, clove, eucalyptus jasmine, patchouli, rose and rosemary.

Common Uses -- Lavender is one of the universal essential oils. It has traditionally been used as a muscle relaxant, soothing agent, skin conditioner and astringent. It is undoubtedly the most versatile and useful of all essential oils. It relaxes, soothes, restores and balances your body and mind. In addition, it calms or stimulates according to your bodies needs. Lavender is excellent for refreshing tired muscles, feet and head. It treats burns and reduces scaring. Can be used neat (undiluted) in small amounts on burns, but care still needs to be taken.

Skin Type -- Sensitive, all skin types

Main Constituents -- Linalol, linalyl acetate, lavandulol, lavandulyl acetate, terpineol, limonene and caryophyllene.

Extraction Method -- solvent extract for the absolute, steam distillation for the essential oil

This page intentionally blank

LEMON

CITRUS LIMON

(Family, Rutaceae*)*

Aromatherapy Class -- Energizing, uplifting

Aroma Type -- Citrus

Perfume Note -- Top

Description -- Lemon trees grow about fifteen feet (five meters) tall. The tree has oval leaves and fragrant white and pale pink flowers with green fruit which turns yellow when mature. Although the tree is native to India and Asia it is now grown in many parts of the world, include North and South America. The essential oil of the lemon tree is derived from the fruit peel, and is penetrating, a little sweet and similar to the smell of lemon juice.

Lemon blends well with bergamot, clary sage, citronella, neroli, orange flower, and violet.

Common Uses -- Lemon has traditionally been used as an antiseptic and soothing agent. It cleanses, refreshes, cools and stimulates. A study conducted in France reported that lemon oil was one of several vaporized essential oil that destroyed 90% of the air-born microbes such as *Streptococcus pyogenes, Proteus,* and *Staphylococcus aureus* within three hours.[10] These antiseptic and bactericidal properties make lemon useful in treating a wide range of respiratory ailments including colds and flu.

Lemon is also useful as an antifungal and has been shown to destroy yeast-like organisms isolated from the human body. In addition, along with eucalyptus, geranium and rose oils, lemon has

---

[10]   Buckle, RGN, J. *Clinical Aromatherapy in Nursing*, San Diego: Singular Publishing, 1997.

been found to be effective in combating *Cryptococcus neoformans* an AIDS-related opportunistic fungus.[11]

Lemon, lavender, tea tree or sweet thyme, diluted in distilled water and applied as a compress can facilitate the mending of broken skin and can be used to irrigate sores and wounds.[12] Lemon is also used to treat oily skin. It is used in skin preparations to tighten the skin and reduce cellulite because of its astringent and toning action on the skin.

Skin Type -- Oily, blemished

Main Constituents -- Limonene, terpinene, pinene, myrcene, citral, linalol, geraniol, citronellal, paracymene (analgesic), bergapten and oxypeucedanin (phototoxic facilitators).

Extraction Method -- Primarily expression however some essential oil is produced by steam distillation.

Safety Information -- Do not use on the skin in direct sunlight. Lemon has a short shelf life (six months).

---

[11] Viollon, c. and J. P. Chaumont. "Antifungal properties of essential oils and their main components upon *Cryptococcus neoformans.*" *Mycopathologia*; 1994, 128(3): 151-153.

[12] Buckle, op cite

ORANGE, SWEET
CITRUS SINENSIS
(Family, Rutaceae)

Aromatherapy Class -- Calming

Aroma Type -- Citrus

Perfume Note -- Top

Description -- Sweet orange should not be confused with bitter orange. Orange essential oil (*citrus aura*ntium) is produced from the fruit of the bitter orange tree and the essential oil neroli is produced from its flowers. Sweet orange (*citrus sinensis*) is produced from the fruit of the sweet orange tree. About thirty grams of essential oil are produced from fifty oranges.

Orange blends well with citrus oils, petitgrain, neroli, and orange flower.

Common Uses -- Orange has traditionally been used as an astringent, a soothing agent and a skin conditioner. It can be used to treat bronchitis and colds, cold sores and to strengthen the immune system. It has also been used traditionally to treat stomach problems, especially those associated with stress and nerves. It normalizes the digestive system, reducing diarrhea and curing constipation.

Orange stimulates the elimination of waste and has been used to treat water retention and PMS. It also reduces the inflammation caused by psoriasis, eczema and other types of dermatitis.

Orange oil is said to help a person achieve emotional equilibrium acting as either a stimulant or sedative, as needed. It also is used to calm the nerves and treat insomnia.

Skin Type -- Dry, aging/mature

Main Constituents -- Limonene, citral, citronellal, geraniol, linalol, perminol, bergapten, auraptenol and acids.

Extraction Method -- Expression

Safety Information -- Do not use on the skin in direct sunlight.

PATCHOULI

POGOSTEMON PATCHOULI

(Family, Lamiaceae [Labiatae])

Aromatherapy Class -- Soothing, toning

Aroma Type -- Woodsy

Perfume Note -- Base

Description -- The essential oil of patchouli is derived from the *pogostemon patchouli* or *Pogostemom cablin* bushes in India, Malaysia and some South American countries. The bush, which grows about three feet tall, has white flowers with a hint of violet. The aroma of the essential oil has been described as being penetrating and potent, earthy and exotic, and sweet and spicy.

Patchouli blends well with bergamot, cedarwood, clary sage, clove, geranium, labdanum, lavender, myrrh, neroli, rose, sandalwood, and vetiver.

Common Uses -- Patchouli has commonly been used as an anti-inflammatory agent, antiseptic, astringent, aphrodisiac, and in perfumes.

Research conducted in India shows that patchouli oil is an effective bactericide against at least 20 Gram-positive and Gram-negative bacteria and 11 yeast-like and filamentous fungi in vitro.[13] Consequently patchouli is valuable for general immune system support. The oil is often used in the East to scent linens and clothes to repel fleas and lice and to help prevent the spread of disease. The sesquiterpene alcohols (patchoulol and bulnesene) in patchouli have moderate anti-microbial effects and also help tone muscles and nerves, and reduce lymphatic and venous congestion.

---

[13]   Pattnaik, S. et al. "Antibacterial and antifunglal activity of ten essential oils in vitro." *Microbios*; 1996, 86(349): 237-246.

Patchouli also possesses anti-inflammatory and cell regenerative (cytophylacitic) properties that make is very useful for general skin care and for treating skin problems like acne, chapped skin, dermatitis, eczema, seborrhea, athlete's foot and dandruff.

Skin Type -- Oily, blemished

Main Constituents -- Patchoulol, pogostol, bulnesol, nor patchoulenol, bulnesene and patchoulene.

Extraction Method -- Steam distillation

PEPPERMINT

MENTHA X PIPERITA

(Family, Lamiaceae [Labiatae])

Aromatherapy Class -- Energizing, stimulating

Aroma Type -- Minty

Perfume Note -- Top

Description -- The peppermint plant produces compact leaves and small white, pink or purple flowers. About 450 kg of plant matter are used to produce 500 grams of clear or yellow essential oil. The distinctive aroma of peppermint oil is extremely refreshing and increases mental clarity and alertness, and sharpens the senses.

Peppermint blends well with bergamot, geranium, lavender, marjoram, rosemary and sandalwood .

Common Uses -- Peppermint is one of the most important essential oils; it has commonly been used as an insect repellent, emollient, antiseptic and muscle relaxant.

The analgesic and antispasmodic properties of peppermint help relieve headache and sinus pain, muscle aches, neuralgia, toothaches and menstrual discomfort. A study conducted at Germany's Neurological Clinic at the University of Kiel demonstrated that the topical application of eucalyptus and peppermint oil to large areas of the forehead and temples produced a muscle-relaxing and mentally relaxing effect. A subsequent study demonstrated that these two oils resulted in a significant temporal muscle-relaxing effect on individuals with experimentally-induced headache pain.[14] This indicates that both oils may be effective in reducing headache pain. Peppermint oil, when applied alone, caused the greatest decrease in participants' sensitivity to headache pain. Both peppermint and eucalyptus oils are well-

---

[14]   Gobel, H., et al. "Effect of peppermint and eucalyptus oil preparations on neurphysiological and experimetnal algesimetric headach parameters." *Cephalagia*; 1994, 14(3): 228-234. ___. "Essential plant oils and headache mechanisms." *Phytomedicine*; 2(2): 93-102.

recognized transmitters in the trigemino-vascular system which is the leading structure in the generation of primary headaches.

Research conducted in India shows that patchouli oil is an effective bactericide against *Escherichia coli* (E. coli) strain SP-11 and at least 22 Gram-positive and Gram-negative bacteria and 11 yeast-like and filamentous fungi in vitro.[15] Peppermint was found to be one of the most effect oils tested against anaerobic oral bacteria[16]. It was also found to be an effective treatment against headlice[17].

Research in Egypt indicates that clove and peppermint essential oils have inhibitory effects on dermatophytic fungi, fungi that cause parasitic skin diseases[18]. Peppermint (and also lemon and eucalyptus) oil has been found to be an effective antibacterial against methicillin-resistant *Staphylococcus aureus* (MRSA)[19]

Peppermint also stimulates, refreshes, cools, restores and uplifts mind and body. It can be included in a massage blend for the digestive system. In addition it is excellent for refreshing tired head and feet.

Skin Type -- Blemished

Main Constituents -- Menthol, carovne, cineol, limonene, menthone, pinene and thymol.

---

[15]   Pattnaik, S. et al. "Effect of essentail oils on the viability and morphology of *Escherichia coli*." *Microbios*; 1995, 84(340): 195-199.

     Pattnaik, S. et al. "Antibacterial and antifunglal activity of ten essential oils in vitro." *Microbios*; 1996, 86(349): 237-246.

[16]   Shapiro, S., et al. "The antimicrobial activity of essential oils and essential oil components towards oral bacteria." *Oral Microbial Immunol*; 1994, 9(4): 202-208. Veal, L. "The potential effectiveness of essential oils as treatment for headlise, Pediculus humanus capitis." *Complement Ther Nurs Midwifery*; 1996, 2(4): 97-101.

[17]   Veal, L. "The potential effectiveness of essential oils as treatment for headlise, Pediculus humanus capitis." *Complement Ther Nurs Midwifery*; 1996, 2(4): 97-101.

[18]   El-Naghy, M. A. et al. "Fungistatic action of natural oils and fatty acids on dermatophytic and saprophytic fungi." *Zentralbl Mikrobiol*; 1992, 147(3-4): 214-220.

[19]   Buckle, RGN, J. *Clinical Aromatherapy in Nursing*, San Diego: Singular Publishing, 1997.

Extraction Method -- Steam distillation

Safety Information -- Can cause skin irritation. Peppermint promotes menstruation and reduces lactation and so should not be used during pregnancy. It should not used with children under the age of 3, or with individuals with epilepsy, insomnia, heart conditions or high blood pressure.

This page intentionally blank

ROSE

ROSA DAMASCENA

(Family, Rosaceae)

Aromatherapy Class -- Cooling, balancing, calming, toning

Aroma Type -- Floral

Perfume Note -- Middle

Description -- There are over 5,000 different varieties of the rose species in the world but only two *Rosa damascena* and *Rosa centifolia* are commonly used to produce essential oils. These are two of the most fragrant of all of the roses. It takes more than 60,000 recently cut roses to produce 30 grams of essential oil. Hence rose is the most expensive of all of the essential oils.

Rose blends well with floral oils, especially jasmine.

Common Uses -- Rose oil is highly prized for skin care because of its astringent, antiseptic and anti-inflammatory properties. It is also virtually non-toxic. Rose has commonly been used to treat emotional shock, general anxiety, insomnia, nervousness, palpitations and stress-related conditions. It has long been held to have mild sedative effects.

Rose is often considered to be a woman's oil because of its ability to help correct female hormone problems; and it has traditionally been used for estrogen support. It promotes and regulates menstruation and relieves the symptoms of PMS. It is also recommended for vaginitis and other uterine and menstrual complaints, frigidity, impotence and sterility.

Rose is a cell regenerator and moisturizer and is helpful for treating slow-healing wounds and scars and for preventing stretchmarks.

Skin Type -- All, especially aging, dry or inflamed skin

Main Constituents -- Rose is a very complex with over 300 different chemical constituents. The primary constitutents are citronellol, geraniol, phenyl ethanol, nerol and stearopten.

Extraction Method -- Steam distillation

Safety Information -- Do not use during the first four months of pregnancy.

ROSEMARY
ROSMARINUS OFFICINALE
(Family, Lamiaceae [Labiatae])

Aromatherapy Class -- Energizing, stimulating

Aroma Type -- Camphoraceous

Perfume Note -- Middle

Description -- The rosemary bush grows almost six feet tall and is covered with small pale blue flowers during the winter months in France, Spain and North Africa. It takes forty-five kilograms of flowers to produce 500 grams of the essential oil. Many feel that the aroma of rosemary from Spain and Northern Africa is similar to the aroma of eucalyptus while rosemary from France smells more like incense.

Rosemary blends well with basil, cedarwood, cinnamon, citronella, lavender, peppermint, and thyme.

Common Uses -- Rosemary has traditionally been used as an antiseptic, muscle relaxant, soothing agent, and skin conditioner. Rosemary has long been used by aestheticians, cosmetologists and dermatologists to rejuvenate hair and skin and to stimulate circulation to the skin and scalp. Research in Europe indicates that a preparation of rosemary, thyme, lavender and cedarwood essential oils in grapeseed and jojoba carrier oils applied topically over a seven month period was an effective treatment for alopecia areata[20,21].

---

[20] Alopecia areata is a common auto-immune disease that results in the loss of hair on the scalp and elsewhere. It usually starts with one or more small, round, smooth patches. It occurs in males and females of all ages and races, but onset most often occurs in childhood. It is estimated that approximately two-percent of the population is affected, or over four million people in the United States. In alopecia areata, the affected hair follicles become very small, drastically slow down production, and grow no hair visible above the surface for months or years. The scalp is the most commonly affected area, but the beard or any hair-bearing site can be affected alone or together with the scalp.

A study conducted in France reported that rosemary oil was one of several vaporized essential oil that destroyed 90% of the air-born microbes such as *Streptococcus pyogenes, Proteus,* and *Staphylococcus aureus* within three hours. Other oils found to be effective were lavender, lemon, peppermint, pine and thyme[22]. Inhalation of the essential oils is effective because the bacteria which cause infections may linger in the sinuses between bouts. These antiseptic and bactericidal properties make rosemary useful in treating a wide range of respiratory ailments including respiratory problems and chest infections.

Rosemary oil is energizing and uplifting, reduces mental fatigue and strain, and enhances memory, thinking and alertness.

Skin Type -- Oily, blemished

Main Constituents -- Borneol, camphene, camphor, cineol, lineol, pinene and terpineol.

Extraction Method -- Steam distillation

Safety Information -- Do not use Rosemary when pregnant, with clients who have high blood pressure, or who suffer from epilepsy. Rosemary may irritate the skin.

---

[21] Hay, I. C. et al. "Randomized trial of aromatherapy. Successful treatment for alopecia areata." *Archive of Dermatology*; 1998, 134(11): 1349-1352.

[22] Buckle, RGN, J. *Clinical Aromatherapy in Nursing*, San Diego: Singular Publishing, 1997.

SANDALWOOD
SANTALUM ALBUM
(Family, Santalaceae)

Aromatherapy Class -- Calming, grounding

Aroma Type -- Woodsy

Perfume Note -- Base

Description -- The sandalwood trees grows up to 27 feet tall (9 meters) over a period of 30 to 64 years. Its yellowish branches are covered with yellow, red or purplish-pink flowers a green leaves. The essential oil is distilled primarily from trees in India. It takes about 11 kilograms of heart-wood to yield 450 to 675 grams of pale yellow or gold oil. The oil has a mild, sweet, and woodsy aroma.

Sandalwood blends well with bergamot, black pepper, clove, geranium, jasmine, labdanum, lavender, mimosa, myrrh, patchouli, rose, violet and vetiver.

Common Uses -- Sandalwood has traditionally been used as an antiseptic, emollient, soothing agent, astringent, insect repellent and skin conditioner.

Tucker[23] reported the results of a study conducted in Japan that showed that the inhalation of sandalwood oil by humans increased alpha-wave activity. This upward shift of brain waves activity is a sign of relaxation. Mice that had been over-agitated by caffeine were sedated by the scent of sandalwood oil. The inhalation of sandalwood, in addition to its sedative effects, is also beneficial for soothing inflammations of the respiratory passages and fighting infections, including dry coughs and bronchitis.

Sandalwood oil is regarded as a hormone regulator and aphrodisiac and is reported to be useful in treating insomnia and impotence.

---

[23]   Tucker, A. "The therapy of aroma." Herbs for Health, 1999, 3(6): 46-50

The sesquiterpene alcohols in sandalwood exert a tonifying effect on muscles and nerves, reduce lymphatic and venous congestion and have moderate anti-microbial properties. It has also been used in Ayurvedic medicine as a remedy for inflammation and eruptive skin disease as an emulsion and paste. Sandalwood is often added to skin treatments for acne and eczema and can be used to sooth sensitive, irritated skin that is cracked or chapped. A recent study also shows that sandalwood has chemopreventive effects and may be an effective agent against skin cancer.[24]

Skin Type -- Oily, blemished, sensitive, and/or dry.

Main Constituents -- Santalols (sesquiterpene alcohol), fusanols, forneol, santalone.

Extraction Method -- Steam distillation

Safety Information -- Sandalwood may cause skin irritations (dermatitis) when applied neat (undiluted).

---

[24]   Dwivedi, C. and A. Abu-Ghazaleh. "Chemopreventive effects of sandalwood oil on skin papillomas in mice." *European Journal of Cancer Prevention*, 1997, 6(4): 399-401.

TEA TREE
AUSTRALIAN *MELALEUCA ALTERNIFOLIA*
(Family, Myrtaceae)

Aromatherapy Class -- Energizing, stimulating, toning

Aroma Type -- Camphoraceous

Perfume Note -- Top

Description -- The tea tree is native to New South Wales and Queensland, Australia. Although there are over 300 varieties of tea tree only one, the *Melaleuca alternifolia*, is used to produce oil for aromtherapy. The camphor-like oil is either clear or pale yellow

Tea Tree blends well with cananga, clary sage, clove, geranium, lavandin, lavender, marjoram, nutmeg and rosemary.

Common Uses -- Tea Tree has traditionally been used as an insect repellent and antiseptic and is know for its remarkable healing qualities. The terpinen-4-ol oil in tea tree is responsible for its germicidal activity and makes it a natural disinfectant, antiseptic and fungicide. Tea tree oil is used by many dentists and doctors to kill germs and prevent the spread of bacteria. It is also a mild analgesic and can even be used as a local anesthetic.

Tea tree oil, according to *The Medical Journal of Australia* is as effective as benzoyl peroxicde in the treatment of acne and provides fewer side effects. It has also been shown to exhibit anti-bacterial and antifungal activity aginst *Candida albicans, Propionibacterium acnes, Pseudomonas aeruginosa, Staphylococcus aureus, Streptococcus pyrogenes, Trichomonas vaginalis,* and *Trichophyton mentagrophytes.* Thus tea tree oil is an effective topical anticeptic for abrasions, bug bites and stings, boils, minor burns, cold sores, cuts and scratches, minor wounds, irritations of the mouth and all types of skin problems. Your first aid kit should include a bottle of tea tree oil.

According to *The Australian Journal of Pharmacy* tea tree oil has been shown to be an effective treatment for mild face and back acne, oral canker sores, non-specific dermatitis and eczema, fungal infections of the fingernails and toenails, herpes simplex outbreaks on the face and lips, infected pustules, and thrush. In addition it is commonly used to treat athlete's foot, chicken pox, itching, lice, poison ivy and oak, ringworm, ulcerous skin conditions, vaginal yeast infections, and warts in Australia.[25]

Skin Type -- Oily, blemished

Main Constituents -- Terpinen-4-ol, cineol, pinene, terpenes, cymene.

Extraction Method -- Steam distillation

Safety Information -- Tea Tree may cause irritation to sensitive skins.

---

[25]   Herb Allure, "Tea Tree Oil." *HART: Herb Allure Resource Toolkit for Nature's Sunshine Products*, 2000.

YLANG YLANG
CANANGA ODORATA
(Family, Annonaceae)

Aromatherapy Class -- Calming, balancing

Aroma Type -- Floral

Perfume Note -- Base/Middle

Description -- The Ylang Ylang tree is tall and slender and covered with large white, pink, yellow or yellow-green flowers. The Malay name "Ylang Ylang" means "flower among flowers" in the Philippines where the tree is native. It is now grown commercially in many tropical regions. About 25 kilograms of recently collected flowers yield 500 grams of the essential oil. This oil is fresh, floral, sweet and seductive. You may also find that it is mildly exciting and exotic like a blend of almond and jasmine.

Ylang Ylang blends well with bergamot, lavender, lemon, narcissus, neroli, palmarosa, sandalwood and vetiver .

Common Uses -- Ylang Ylang has traditionally been used in perfume and as an aphrodisiac. However, it is also used as a sedative and relaxant and has been applied to reduce high blood pressure, and to normalize cardiopulmonary rhythms. Only a small amount applied topically is needed to have a significant effect.

The antispasmodic and antifungal effects of Ylang ylang are due to his ester content. In addition, the sesquiterpene caryophyllene in Ylang ylang provide anti-inflammatory and bactericidal effects. The borneol in Ylang ylang exhibits anti-acethylcholine activity and thus may also be used as an anti-emetic (acethlcholine is a neurotransmitter which stimulates vomiting).

Skin Type -- Oily, dry, normal to combination, aging/mature

Main Constituents -- Methyl benzoats, methyl salicylate, linalyl acetate, cadinene, caryophyllene, pinene, cresol, eugenol, linalol, geraniol, and borneol.

Extraction Method -- Solvent extraction

Safety Information -- Ylang ylang possesses opiate-like properties which provide analgesic effects. However it may enhance the effect of opiate drugs like morphine and codeine. In addition, heavy use may cause headaches.

Seven
Carrier Oils

This chapter introduces some of the more common carrier oils. Essential oils can be used full strength (that's call using them "neat") but usually they are diluted in carrier oil. Theoretically any vegetable oil could be used as a carrier. However different carrier oils have different properties so you should use as much care in selecting carrier oils as you do in selecting essential oils. Never use mineral oil as a carrier oil. Mineral oil is a petroleum product and your body was not meant to be covered in petroleum. Mineral oil molecules are so large that they can not penetrate the skin and, rather than facilitating the absorption of the essential oils, will impede essential oil absorption.

As noted above, carrier oils should be vegetable oils. In addition, they should be fresh and without odor. You don't want the smell of the carrier oil to overpower the scent of the essential oils. The carrier oil should be cold pressed and without chemical additives. If possible, select carrier oil which is certified organic. Most vegetable oils will go rancid fairly quickly. When you are mixing an essential oil with carrier oil you may want to add drops of Vitamin E from a vitamin capsule to the oil. The Vitamin E will help preserve the carrier oil and is good for the skin. If you do decide to add Vitamin E makes sure that it is organic, some of the Vitamin E sold in stores in produced in laboratories.

The carrier oils presented in this chapter are:

- Almond
- Avocado
- Canola
- Jojoba
- Olive
- Peanut
- Sun flower
- Wheat germ

Almond Oil
Prunus amygdalus var. dulcis

Contents   Glucosides, minerals, rich in protein, vitamins A, B1, B2, B6 and E

Uses   Helpful for all skin types. Especially good for eczema. helps relieve itching, soreness, dryness and inflammation Useful against burns and thread veins. Very lubricating, but not penetrating, which makes it a good massage oil and protectant. Almond oil rapidly goes rancid so use blend made with it quickly. It can be used 100% strength.

Avocado Oil
Persea americana

Contents   Protein, lecithin, fatty acids, vitamins A. B1, B2, Pantothenic acid (B5), D, E

Uses   Avocado oil is very penetrating. It is good for nourishing dry and dehydrated skin, eczema, solar kurtosis, and it improves elasticity. It is a very thick heavy oil and so is best blended with other carrier oils. Also, it is a very long-lasting oil.

Canola Oil
Brassica napus/campestris

Contents   Minerals, high GLA, vitamins

Uses   Canola oil is odorless, and very stable. It penetrates the skin very quickly and is used for all skin types. Being very light it is useful for massage. It is a long-lasting oil that resists rancidity.

Jojoba Oil
Simmondsia californica

Contents   Protein, minerals, plant wax, myristic acid.

Uses   Jojoba oil mimics sebum and penetrates skin very rapidly. Therefore it is not good for massage but is excellent for nourishing the skin. It is used for healing for inflamed skin, psoriasis, eczema, and any sort of dermatitis. It can help control acne and oily skin or scalp because excess sebum actually dissolves in jojoba. It is an anti-oxidant and may help extend the life of other oils. It is used for hair care and for all skin types. However, it can clog pores. Myristic acid is anti-inflammatory, so Jojoba oil is a good base oil for treating rheumatism and arthritis. Jojoba is the favorite carrier oil of most aromatherapists.

Other observations   Jojoba is *not* an oil, it is a wax which is liquid at room temperature. The wax is found on the inside of the jojoba seed, a seed that looks a lot like a coffee bean. Jojoba is the only naturally occurring monoglyceride from a non-animal source. That is pretty amazing because there are over 300,000 plants that produce some form of oil.

All other seed oils are triglycerides. The triple strand of triglycerides has an anchor-like shape. This shape makes it hard, if not impossible, for the oil molecules to penetrate the pores of the human skin. The structure of the jojoba molecule, a monoglyceride, is snake-like which moves easily through the pores of the skin and doesn't leave an oily surface. Consequently jojoba helps the skin retain moisture but does not prevent the transpiration of toxins and gases through the skin.

Researchers at the University of Arizona discovered in 1933 that the molecular structure of jojoba is very similar to that of our own skin oil. It is almost impossible to find someone who reacts negatively to jojoba oil because of this similarity. In addition, jojoba dissolves sebum, the waxy material left behind when our subacueous glands produce oil to moisturize our skin. Sebum clogs pores and suffocates hair follicles on the head and eyelashes resulting in one form of hair loss and breakage. Thus jojoba oil should be used as the carrier any time you are preparing a blend to treat oily skin or skin problems like acne.

Olive Oil

Olea europaea

Contents   Vitamins, protein, minerals,

Uses   Olive oil has a relatively strong odor that makes it more useful with strongly scented essential oils. It is used to help treat rheumatic conditions, for hair care and cosmetics, and for nail and hair care. It is helpful for inflamed or acne skin and for treating bruises and sprains. It has traditionally been used to produce macerated oils.

Peanut Oil

Arachis hypogeae

Contents   Protein, vitamins, minerals

Uses   Peanut oil is good for all skin types and as an emollient for arthritis or sunburn. Normally it is used as an additive because of its strong odor. It is a heavy oil that penetrates the skin slowly and so it is good for massage. Peanut oil is not especially long lasting and so should be used quickly.

Other observations   SOME PEOPLE ARE EXTREMELY ALLERGIC TO THIS OIL. PERFORM A PATCH TEST BEFORE USING.

Sunflower Oil

Helianthus annuus

Contents   Vitamins A, B,D, E, minerals, lecithin, inulin,, high in unsaturated fatty acids.

Uses   Sunflower oil is good for all skin types, and is used to treat leg ulcers and skin diseases, bruises, diaper rash, and cradle cap. It is easily absorbed and has a light textured. Sunflower oil is often used as a carrier oil.

Wheat germ Oil

Contents   Protein, minerals, vitamins E, A & D

Uses   Wheat germ oil is often used to help treat dry cracked skin, eczema, psoriasis, prematurely aged skin, stretch marks. It is a thick, sticky oil and some sources say it is an anti-oxidant. Because it is thick it should be used in a 10% dilution with another carrier oil.

Other observations   Wheat Germ Oil can be very dangerous for a person with a severe wheat or gluten allergy or gluten sensitivity, like Celiac disease, or the associated disease, dermatitis herpitiformus. Both diseases are sensitive to the gluten in the wheat germ, and it might inadvertently be absorbed through the skin.

Eight

An Introduction to Blending, and Methods of Application

There are several topics that need to be addressed before we look at methods of blending and applying essential oils. The first is essential oil safety.

Essential Oil Safety

Care should be taken when using essential oils in the following situations or with clients who have the following medical conditions.

1. *Cancer* Potentially carcinogenic oils like basil, tarragon, and yellow and brown camphor should not be used with cancer clients. Anise, fennel, star anise and other hormonal oils should not be used with clients who have estrogen-dependent cancers.

2. *Children* Essential oils should not be used on premature babies or newborns and peppermint should not be used with children. All essential oils should be kept out of the reach of small children.

3. *Diabetes* Diabetics should not use angelica.

4. *Epilepsy* It is well documented that any powerful smell can initiate an epileptic attack. Therefore when working with a client with epilepsy the use of essential oils with strong aromas like camphor, eucalyptus, fennel, hyssop, lavandin, lavender, peppermint, rosemary, sage, (all types) tea tree, thyme, yarrow and wormwood should be avoided.

5. *Heart Disease* Peppermint and cornmint should not be used with clients who suffer from heart conditions.

6. *High or low blood pressure* I have not been able to find any published, scientific studies which report on the effect of blood pressure changes following the external application of essential

oils on humans.   However several herbs have been used traditionally to treat blood pressure and heart conditions and consequently should not be used with clients who have blood pressure problems or heart conditions. Clove, Hyssop, Juniper, Spike Lavender, Peppermint and Thymol and wild Thyme should not be used with clients who have high blood pressure.

7. ***Hypoglycemia*** is caused by the excess production of insulin by the Pancreas gland causing blood sugar levels to drop, often to dangerously low levels.   Individuals who are hypoglycemic should avoid Geranium because it reduces blood sugar levels and can cause symptoms of hypoglycemia.

8. ***Photosensitization*** (sometimes referred to as phototoxicity) occurs when a substance coming into contact with the skin can react with ultra violet light. This reaction can cause anything from mild brown blotches through to severe burning of the skin. The condition can be very long lasting and any time the skin is exposed to ultra violet light the condition can recur. It is vital to remember that it is ultra violet light that causes the problem and this can occur even on relatively dull days. Bergamot is one of the main essential oil to avoid with individuals who are photosensitive.   Other citruses like grapefruit, lemon, and lime may also cause photosensitivity.

9. ***Pregnancy*** Most concerns about essential oil use during pregnancy arise from the traditional use of water-soluble herbal extracts when taken internally.   Such extracts may be very different from essential oil of the same plant, especially when the essential oil is administered externally.   Nevertheless, care should be taken when using essential oils with a pregnant woman and prudence dictates that when in doubt the use of a questionable essential oil should be avoided. One of the main contra-indications of essential oils use during pregnancy is the heightened chance of causing skin irritation (see below). It is quite common in late pregnancy for the skin to become very itchy and sometimes inflamed. In such circumstances essential oils in massage or bath might aggravate the condition.   In addition, emmenagogues, hormonal oils and neurotoxic oils should not be used during pregnancy and no essential oils should be used during the first trimester if there is any danger of miscarriage.   Essential oils should not be used vaginally or

rectally by pregnant women. Consequently oils which should not be used during pregnancy include: Angelica root, Basil, Birch, Carrot, Cedarwood, Chamomile, Cinnamon, Citus, Citronella, Clove, Coriander, Cypress, Eucalyptus, (except Eucalyptus, smithii), Fennel, Fir, Frankincense, Geranium, Helichrysum, Juniper, Lavandin, Lavender, Lemongrass, Marjoram, Melissa, Myrrh, Myrtle, Narde, Niaouli, Oregano, Peppermint, Scotch Pine, Ravensara, Rose, Rosemary, Clary Sage, Tea Tree, Thyme, Vetiver, Wintergreen and Yarrow.

10.*Skin Irritation* occurs when some substance comes into contact with the skin, and causes anything from a mild itch to burns. Once the substance is removed and healing takes place, there should be no more problems.

11.*Skin Sensitization* occurs when a substance has been introduced to the skin and it causes a permanent change in the immune system in a similar manner to a vaccination. This is a much more serious problem than skin irritation because once the body has been sensitized a reaction may occur the next time the same or a similar substance is used. The reaction can range from a mild itch to anaphylactic shock. However, the later is almost unknown in aromatherapy. If an irritating or burning sensation or a blotchy irritable skin rash are noticed then that particular oil or chemically similar ones should not be used again.

As you practice aromatherapy and work with essential oils you will develop your understanding of when and how to use and not use specific essential oils. We use a client in-take form (Appendix A) with our clients. Among other things the in-take form asks about medical conditions which may require aromatherapy treatment or for which we need to be cautious.

Essential Oil Measurement

As you become more involved in aromatherapy you will discover that there are many different ways of measuring essential oils: milliliters and ounces, teaspoons and tablespoons, and drops and percentages. You need to learn how to measure essential oils for proper dilution to use them safely and effectively. Essential oils are measured by volume and not by weight. Different essential oils have different densities so the same volume of two different essential oils may have different weights. Thus the measures below are volume not weight measures.

We will use the following abbreviations:

- ml = milliliters
- oz = fluid ounce
- tsp = teaspoon
- TBS = tablespoon
- gtts = drops (the use of this abbreviation is not universal)[26]

Here are a few equivalencies between the different measures:

- 1 ml = 20 drops
- 1 oz = 30 ml [27]
- 1 tsp = 5 ml
- 1 tsp = 100 drops
- 1 TBS = 3 tsp
- 1 TBS = 15 ml
- 1 TBS = 1/2 oz
- 1 TBS = 300 drops
-

When we mix oils we usually want to achieve a specific percentage dilution. For example, a 5% dilution is one in which the essential oils make up 5% of the solution and the carrier oils the other 95%. Here are a few rules of thumb for mixing oils. These are not exact but very close and even better, they are easy to remember and use. The method that we are going to use below is an approximation but it works well when small quantities of oil are being mixed. If you need to be exact then use a one ml pipette (serological pipette) graduated to tenths or hundredths of a ml.

---

[26]   If you have studied Spanish then you might recall that a drop is a *gota* and that a little drop is a *gotita.* Little drops in Spanish are *gotitas,* similar to gtts.

[27]   For the purists a British fluid ounce is 28.412 ml, an American fluid ounce is 29.573 ml.

Table 1

Essential Oil Measurements

Percentage Dilution	Drops of Essential Oil	Measure of Carrier Oil
5%	5	5 ml
2%	2	5 ml
1%	1	5 ml

Now let's try a few practical problems.

1.   Suppose that you want to mix a 5% dilution of massage oil using 3 TBS of carrier oil. How many drops of essential oil would you need to add to the carrier oil?

_____ Drops

Solution:

It is hard to multiply or add TBS and gtts so let's begin by converting the 3 TBS into gtts so that we are thinking in terms of gtts. Multiply 3 TBS by the number of drops per tablespoon:

$$3 \text{ TBS (300 gtts per TBS)} = 900 \text{ gtts}$$

Now we can compute 5% of 900 gtts:

$$0.05 \ (900 \text{ gtts}) = 45 \text{ gtts}^{28}$$

So, you need to add **45 drops** (gtts) of essential oil to 3 TBS (or 900 gtts) of carrier oil to have a 5% dilution.

2.   You want to prepare one ounce of a 3% dilution. How many drops of essential oil should you add to the ounce of carrier oil?

---

28   Remember that 5% = 5/100 = 0.05

_____ Drops

Solution:

Again, let's begin by converting the carrier oil measure into drops. From the conversion table on the previous page you can see that one ounce is equal to 30 ml and that 1 ml is equal to 20 gtts. Multiply 30 ml by 20 drops per ml. So one ounce is equivalent to 600 drops:

$$1 \text{ ounce} = 30 \text{ ml}$$

$$30 \text{ ml}(20 \text{ gtts per ml}) = 600 \text{ gtts}$$

Now we can multiply the number of drops of carrier oil times the percentage dilution that we want to get the needed number of drops of essential oil:

$$0.03 \ (600 \text{ gtts}) = 18 \text{ gtts}$$

So, you would need to add 18 drops of essential oil to the 1 ounce of carrier oil to mix a 3% dilution.

3.   A recipe calls for 2 TBS of carrier oil and 12 drops of essential oil. What is the essential oil dilution in the recipe?

_____ %

Solution:

Once again, let's begin by converting the 2 TBS of carrier oil into the equivalent number of drops. Again we need to multiply 2 TBS by 300 drops per tablespoon:

$$2 \text{ TBS} (300 \text{ gtts per TBS}) = 600 \text{ gtts}$$

Now we can divide the number of drops of essential oil by the number of drops of carrier oil to compute the dilution percentage:

$$\text{Dilution Percentage} = 12 \text{ gtts} / 600 \text{ gtts} = 0.02 = 2\%$$

So, the recipe results in a 2 percent essential oil dilution.

Blending Essential Oils

The first step in blending essential oils is to carefully identify the desired effects and/or the condition that you want to treat. Only after you have done this should you select the essential oils. It is important to identify the intended use of the essential oils first so that you don't select essential oils that have counteracting effects. For example, you normally would not combine a stimulant like peppermint with a sedative or relaxant like chamomile.

You may decide to use one essential oil in a carrier oil. However most aromatherapists strive for a synergistic effect by combining two to five essential oils with a carrier. Using more than five essential oils is usually not recommended because, as you add more essential oils to a blend, the possibility of including essential oils with counteracting affects increases.

As you begin blending essential oils you will probably use equal proportions in your blends. With more experience you will start to use a higher percentage of one essential oil, because of its desired properties, and proportionately less of others.

The Table 2 below identifies common essential oil uses; the suggested total number of drops of essential oil (EO); and when appropriate, the quantity of carrier oil to be used.

Blending Perfumes

Perfumes are designed by mixing different essential oils. However, in the commercial perfume industry chemical substitute oils are usually used for all, except the most expensive, perfumes. Essential oils are divided into three categories for perfume blending: bottom notes, middle notes, and top notes. Top note oils are the first oils that you sense when you smell a perfume. They are also are the first to dissipate in the air and lose their influence. Bottom notes are the aromas that linger for a long time. They may not be perceptible at first but they last and provide the base for the perfume. Middle notes, as their name implies, are in the middle.

Table 2
Common Essential Oil Uses

Use	EO	Base
Bath oil	8 to 10 drops	Warm bath water in a bathtub
Body lotion	15 to 20 drops	1 ounce of unscented base lotion (use a vegetable base lotion)
Clay facial mask	2 to 5 drops	2 tablespoons of powdered clay mixed with distilled water or other desired liquid
Clay partial body pack	5 drops per 1/4 cup of clay	1/4 to 1/2 cup of powdered clay mixed with distilled water or other desired liquid
Facial oil	3 to 5 drops	1/2 ounce of carrier oil
Inhalation	2 to 5 drops	Clean tissue
Massage oil	10 to 20 drops	1 ounce of carrier oil
Skin tonic spritzer	20 to 30 drops	4 ounces of distilled water
Steam facial or inhalation	5 to 10 drops	Bowl of hot water

When blending perfumes always start with the base note, then add middle notes and finish with top notes. You may recall that the essential oil profiles identified the note of each oil. Table 3 below will help you blend.

Table 3
Essential Oil Notes

Bottom Notes	Middle Notes	Top Notes
Angelica	Chamomile	Bergamot
Cedarwood	Clary Sage	Cardamon
Frankincense	Cypress	Eucalyptus
Jasmine	Geranium	Grapefruit
Myrrh	Ginger	Lemon
Patchouli	Lavender	Lemongrass
Sandalwood	Juniper	Lime
Tuberose	Neroli	Mandarin
Vanilla	Palmarosa	Tangerine
Vetiver	Rose	Tea Tree
	Rosemary	Orange (Sweet)
	Rosewood	
	Ylang Ylang	

To give you an idea of how professional perfumers blend perfumes review the table below of some popular fragrances. As you review the composition of these different perfumes, think about how the blenders have used top, middle and base notes.

Table 4
Popular Perfume Oils

Fragrance	Contents
Arabesque	floral, musk, sandalwood, herb
Chanel No. 19	iris, jasmine, rose, ylang ylang, French moss, musk. sandalwood
Chantilly	orange blossom, spice, chypre, sandalwood, vetiver, patchouli

Chloé	vetiver, oak moss, patchouli, jasmine, musk, tuberose
Givenchy III	amber, musk
Halston	jasmine
Jontue	jasmine, tuberose, honeysuckle, jonquil
Joy	rose absolute, jasmine absolute
Mackie	jasmine, rose, jonquil
Shalimar	patchouli, vanilla, bergamot, iris
Tabu	rose, jasmine, musk, amber
V'E Versace	ylang ylang, lily, Bulgarian rose
White Shoulders	violet, rose, tuberose, jasmine
Y	ylang ylang

Sample Blends

This section presents some of our favorite therapeutic massage blends. You can use them as examples to help develop your own blends or try them as they are.

Respiratory Therapy

1 oz carrier oil (2 TBS)

10 drops Geranium oil

8 drops Peppermint oil

5 drops Rosemary oil

Cellulite Fighter

1 oz carrier oil

10 drops Geranium oil

10 drops Juniper oil

5 drops Pink Grapefruit oil

3 drops Rosemary oil

5 drops Thyme Oil

3 drops Vetiver oil

PMS Relief

1 oz carrier oil

10 drops Clary sage oil

10 drops Geranium oil

5 drops Nutmeg oil

3 drops Rose Bulgaria oil

Muscle and Joint Pain Relief

1 oz carrier oil

8 drops Clove Bud oil

6 drops Ginger oil

4 drops Nutmeg oil

Clear the Mind

1 oz carrier oil

8 drops Basil oil

6 drops Lavender oil

4 drops Pink Grapefruit oil

4 drops Rosemary oil

Immune System Therapy

1 oz carrier oil

7 drops Lavender oil

5 drops Ravensara oil

7 drop Roman Chamomile oil

5 drops Tea Tree oil

Romance Enhancer

1 oz carrier oil

8 drops Jasmine absolute

6 drops Rose Bulgaria oil

3 drops Sandalwood oil

3 drops Ylang Ylang oil

Calm the Spirit Blend

1 oz carrier oil

8 drops Bergamot oil

4 drops Geranium oil

6 drops Neroli oil

6 drops Roman Chamomile oil

4 drops Rose Bulgaria oil

There are many different ways to use essential oils. It may seem at first that the only way to use them is to prepare massage oils but there are a lot of different ways to enjoy and benefit from essential oils. We hope that you will try and enjoy the following.

Lavender Body Lotion

1/4 tsp. borax

1 tsp. white beeswax

1 tsp. lanolin

2 TBS vegetable glycerin

5 tsp. apricot kernel oil

4 tsp. cold-pressed sunflower oil

20 drops Lavender oil

Preparation Instructions

1. Dissolve the borax in 2 TBS of boiled water
2. Melt the beeswax, lanolin and vegetable glycerin with the apricot and sunflower oils in a double boiler. Remove from heat once the wax has melted
3. Add the borax solution and mix well. The lotion should turn white and thicken. Keep mixing until cool.
4. Stir in the Lavender oil
5. Pour into a glass jar and store in a cool, dark place.

Variation: Use 10 drops of Peppermint oil in place of the Lavender oil for a refreshing and invigoration lotion.

Body Scrub

2 TBS powdered orange rind

3 TBS ground almonds

2 TBS oatmeal

1 tsp. red rose petals

6 TBS almond oil

5 drops lavender (or other flower oil like jasmine, rose or neroli)

5 drops sandalwood (or other wood oil like cedar or rosewood)

Preparation Instructions

1. Blend all of the dry ingredients together
2. Add the almond oil one tablespoon at a time and blend into a crumbly paste.
3. Stir in the essential oils
4. Store in a glass jar and use within two weeks

Moisture Cream

1/2 Cup rosewater (look for it in your local health food store)

1/2 tsp. Glycerin

2 TBS witch hazel (look for it in your local health food store)

1/2 tsp. Borax (cleaning section in your supermarket)

2 TBS white bee's wax

1 tsp. Lanolin (look for it in your local health food store)

2 TBS almond oil

2 drops rose oil

Preparation Instructions

1. Gently heat the rosewater, glycerin, witch hazel and borax in a glass or stainless steel saucepan until the borax has dissolved.

2. Melt the bee's wax, lanolin and almond oil together in a double boiler over low heat.

3. When the bee's wax has melted, slowly add the rosewater mixture to the bee's wax mixture, whisking as you do so. The mixture will thicken quickly.

4. Remove from heat and continue to whisk until it cools.

5. Add the rose oil.

6. Pour the cream into glass jars and store.

Hand Cream for Dry or Chapped Skin

3 oz. unscented, hard, white soap

4 oz. white bee's wax

3 TBS Glycerin

2/3 Cup almond oil

3 TBS rosewater

25 drops patchouli oil

Preparation Instructions

1. Grate the soap and place it in a bowl. Add 6 TBS boiling water and stir until the mixture is smooth.

2. Combine the bee's wax, almond oil, rosewater and glycerin in a double boiler. Melt over low heat.

3. Remove from heat when bee's wax has melted and gradually stir in the soap mixture. Keep stirring until the mixture is cool.

4. Add the patchouli drops and mix well.

5. Pour into wide mouth glass jars

As we hope that you have noted, there are lots of wonderful ways to use essential oils. Experiment and have lots of fun.

Nine
The Business of Aromatherapy

Congratulations, you are well on your way to becoming an aromatherapist. You might be thinking now about a part-time or full-time career in aromatherapy. It is an exciting health-related field with lots of opportunities. This unit is designed to help you take the next steps in your career as an aromatherapist.

Finding Your Niche

Before you start working as an aromatherapist it is a good idea to do a little market research. This will help you determine the level and type of demand which exists for aromatherapy services in your community, and the level of competition.

Start by trying to answer the following questions:

1. What are the characteristics of the people who will want aromatherapy services?

2. How many people that demonstrate these characteristics live in my market area?

3. How many other professional aromatherapists are there in my market area?

4. How much would potential clients be willing to pay for my services?

5. How many times or how frequently would a client want my services?

6. Are there other holistic healthcare professionals in my market area with whom I could build professional links? If so, who are they?

One study, conducted in England, indicated that seventy-five percent of all people who use alternative healthcare services are age 45 or over, that sixty-five percent of them are women and that they usually visit an alternative healthcare provider three times. Thus you might expect that your primary market consists of middle-aged and older women and men and that you can expect some repeat business.

You can quickly discover how much competition you may experience by checking the yellow pages in the telephone directory. After identifying the competition it would be a good idea to visit at least a few aromatherapists to discover what services they provide and how much they charge for their services. Don't forget that some licensed massage therapists also offer aromatherapy treatments.

Identify and then make contact with other holistic healthcare practitioners in your market area. These practitioners might include naturopaths, massage therapists, chiropractors, osteopaths, physical therapists, acupuncturists and health food/herbal stores. Offer to refer clients to them when appropriate and/or place their brochures in your office in exchange for the same.

Once you have analyzed the market you will need to think about where you would like to practice and whether to work full time or part time. You may decide to work on an "on call" basis out of your home, rent space in a clinic or massage studio, or rent or buy your own clinic. You also may decide to work as a sole practitioner or work with or for another aromatherapist. These decisions are important because they will affect your future business decisions.

Selecting Your Tools

Your primary tools as an aromatherapist are your knowledge of essential oils and their uses and your hands. Nevertheless, you will need to purchase a few other tools as well. Because many of your aromatherapy treatments will be applied to the skin (massage) you will need a good massage table. We suggest that you purchase a portable massage table so that you can take it with you to visit clients if necessary. You can usually find a good entry-level massage table on the Internet for about $150. You will find many reliable sources for tables and massage equipment on the internet. Of course you will also need massage table sheets and towels.

Basic Massage Table

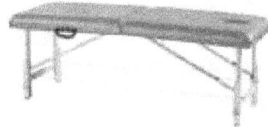

You will also need to find one or more reliable sources for essential oils and base oils. Again, check the internet for vendors and prices. Once you have a tax number or a resale number you can purchase oils at wholesale prices which can be as low as 50% of the retail list price.

Deciding which essential oils to purchase for your self or to stock can be tricky business with about 300 essential oils to choose from. You have studied some of the most important basic essential oils. The following is a list of Frontier Natural Products Co-op's best-selling essential oils. It will give you an idea of which oils are most popular among consumers.

Lavender (Lavandula angustifolia)--floral, sweet, herbaceous. Used for balancing, calming and normalizing.

Eucalyptus (Eucalyptus globules)--camphoraceous. Used for purifying, invigorating and cooling.

Peppermint (Mentha piperita)--minty, sharp. Used for vitalizing, refreshing and cooling.
Tea Tree (Melaleuca alternifolia)--camphoraceous. Used for cleansing, purifying and uplifting.

Patchouli (Pogostemon cablin)--earthy, herbaceous, sweet, balsamic, woody. Used for soothing, it is exotic and sensual.

Sandalwood (Santalum album)--soft, woody, sweet, earthy, balsamic, tenacious. Used for relaxing and centering, it is exotic and sensual.

Rosemary (Rosmarinum officinalis)--herbaceous, camphorous, woody, balsamic with evergreen undertones. Used for clarifying, warming and invigorating.

Ylang ylang (Cananga odorata)--sweet, floral, heavy, tropical, with spicy-balsamic undertones. This oil is romantic, exotic and alluring.

Geranium (Pelargonium graveolens)--sweet, green, citrus-rose and fresh. Used for balancing and normalizing.

Clove bud (Syzygium aromaticum)--spicy, sweet and warm. Used for warming and sense enhancing.

Although you can use cotton for essential oil inhalation you should also consider purchasing a diffuser. A diffuser suitable for use in a normal sized room should cost less than $100.

You may also want to expand your services to include product sales. If so, consider stocking essential oil-based hydrosols, creams and lotions, gels, soaps, and shampoos. You may also want to stock diffusers, dispersing agents, base oils and essential oils.

Marketing and Pricing Your Services

You *must* develop a marketing plan if you are going to have a successful aromatherapy business, or any other business for that matter. If you don't have a marketing plan and don't market then whatever you are doing is just a hobby. The plan does not need to be and lengthy, impressive, bound document and you don't need to hire a consultant to develop it for you. In fact, it is better if you do it yourself.

Your marketing plan should answer the following seven key questions:

1. What is the purpose of your business?

2. How will I achieve this purpose?

3. What is the identity of my business?

4. What is my market niche?

5. Who are the members of my target market?

6. What are the marketing weapons that I will use?

7. How much, as a percentage of gross revenue, will I spend on marketing?

The first question helps you define the purpose of your business. If you don't know why you are in business and what your business has to offer it will be hard to convince potential clients that you can help them. The answer to the first question may be something like: "The Aromatherapy Studio provides the highest quality personalized aromatherapy treatment at a competitive price."

The second question helps you crystallize in your own mind the services and products that you plan to offer. For example, you may write: "This will be achieved by offering full-body aromatherapy massages, inhalation treatment, essential oil foot reflexology, and an aroma bar." This part of your plan should identify your competitive advantages and benefits . . . identify what you do that is different from the services provided by your competitors.

Your answer to the third question defines your business's identity. The identity of your business is not its "image". A business image is an artificial projection . . . it tells potential clients "This is what we *want* you to think that we are." Your image tells your clients and potential clients what you *really* are. An identity is honest and that is important because clients, with the passage of time, will not discover that your business is different from what you say that it is. We want you to think hard about your business's identity so we are not going to give you a sample answer to this question.

Your answers to questions four and five should be related. Your nitch is your position in the marketplace. Your nitch might be alternative healthcare services, it might be the relaxation market or it might be sports ("weekend warriors" get hurt and need aromatherapy treatments too). Once you have defined your position in the market then identify the people who are consumers in that nitch . . . the answer to question five. These are the people to whom you want to direct your marketing messages.

There are many marketing weapons available. Select those that you think you can use effectively. Weapons typically used by small businesses include:

- ✓ Booths at the county fair
- ✓ Brochures
- ✓ Business cards
- ✓ Canvassing

✓ Circulars (single sheet printed material, less complex than a brochure)
✓ Classified ads
✓ Direct mail
✓ Free seminars
✓ Magazine ads
✓ Newsletter (traditional and web-site based)
✓ Newspaper display ads
✓ On-line classified add (check out banner exchange programs)
✓ Personal letters
✓ Radio spots
✓ Signs (outdoor and indoor)
✓ Signs on bulletin boards
✓ TV spots (check out your local cable company and see if they have a low cost channel)
✓ Web site
✓ Yellow pages

Finally, decide how much you can afford and want to *invest* in marketing. Don't think of marketing as an expense, think of it as an investment in the future of your business. However, don't invest in more marketing weapons that you can successfully use.

Pricing

Pricing will affect the demand for your services. Two approaches to pricing are (1) market-based pricing and (2) cost-based pricing. You should use a combination of the two. In market-based pricing you do a little research, call competitors for example, and find out how much they charge for similar or identical services. The internet is great for this kind of research because many aromatherapy studios and stores have opened web sites and you can check their prices very quickly. Remember to adjust their prices for regional pricing differences. For example the prices for services at a studio in New York City will be higher, maybe much higher, than what you could charge in a small mid-Western town.

The second approach to pricing is to base your prices on the cost of your services. For example you may identify the following costs for a one-hour whole body massage:

Your time	$30.00	(Pay yourself first)
Carrier oil	$ 1.00	
Essential oils	$ 3.00	
Total	$33.00	

But wait! Are those all of your costs? What about the $500 per month rent that you pay? What about your $150 per month electricity bill and the $50 per month for the phone? Oh, and then there are the eight sheets for the massage table, they cost $30 each and you have to clean them after each use. These costs are called overhead or indirect costs and they are just as important as the direct costs listed above.

Let's assume that you think that you will provide four hours of service per day, 20 days per month. In that case then each hour of service must also cover $6.25 of the rent ($500/80 hours of services). Each hour of service must also cover the costs of the utilities and telephone. Those costs per hour of service are $1.88 for electricity ($150/80) and $0.63 for telephone ($50/80 hours). Assume that you think that you will have to replace the massage table sheets every six months and that it costs an average of $0.25 to clean each sheet. The total cost of the sheets was $240 and over six months you plan on giving 480 massages (4 massages per day, 20 days per month, 6 months). The cost per massage per sheet is $0.50 ($240 / 480 massages), you need to include the replacement cost of the sheets in your price each time you give a massage; and don't forget the cleaning cost. Now let's see what our cost is for a one-hour massage:

Table 1
Cost Calculation

Your time	$30.00	(Pay yourself first)
Carrier oil	$ 1.00	
Essential oils	$ 3.00	
Rent	$ 6.25	
Utilities	$ 1.88	
Telephone	$ 0.63	
Sheets	$ 0.75	(Prorated replacement cost plus cleaning cost)
Total Cost	$43.51	

We just added $8.25 to the cost of a massage, and to the amount that you need to charge to cover all of your expenses. Did we include all of the expenses? No, probably not. You should include your investment in advertising and you may have other expenses as well, like insurance and taxes.

The next step in cost-based pricing, after you have quantified all of the costs, is to multiply the cost by your profit percentage to compute your service price. Assume that you want to earn a profit equal to 20% of your costs and that the cost of a one-hour aromatherapy massage is $42.25 as we computed above.

The price of the one-hour aromatherapy massage would be computed as:

Price = Cost (1+profit percentage)
Price = $43.51 (1 + 0.20)
Price = $43.51 (1.20)
Price = $52.21

Now you are ready to compare your price with that of your competition. If there is a big difference between your price and that of your competition then ask yourself why. For example, if your price is significantly less than that of your competition then are you just lucky and you have lower costs? Or, did you forget to include some other costs? If your price is significantly higher have your overestimated costs? Is the competition more efficient? If so, why? What costs can you reduce or eliminate?

Pricing is critical to the long-term success of your business. If your prices are too low it may be hard for you to stay in business over the long term. If your prices are too high you may lose clients to lower-priced competitors. Find a profitable balance and enjoy your business.

Getting Started

Now that you know what you want to do, do it! Purchase your supplies and materials, start advertising, get the necessary licenses and permits and make a plan to open your business. It may be part time in a spare room in your house of full time in a strip mall. In any case, make a plan and follow it.

Scorekeeping

Scorekeeping has two aspects, marketing and financial. Review your marketing plan to identify the weapons that are working well and those that are not effective. Drop the ones that are not effective and transfer the money that you were spending on them to the weapons that are effective.

Keep track of your revenues and expenses and monitor your costs. That information will be critical to determining the profitability of your aromatherapy business and to identifying the profitable products and services. Modify your product and service mix to maintain profitability.

You should think about hiring an accountant or purchasing accounting software. Both will make record keeping much easier and will ensure that you have the information that you need to make wise business decisions.

Conclusion

Whether you do aromatherapy for yourself, your family or as a business it can change your life. You can take the essence of nature with you wherever you go with your essential oils. Essential oils heal with the power of nature. The complex chemical compositions of natural essential oils have demonstrated healing properties. We believe that natural essential oils do even more. Our souls remember through sounds, especially music, and smells. You may discover that essential oils heal not only the body but also the soul.

Resources

You can support your local business by purchasing essential oils and herbal products from a local health store. If you can't find what you need or want to purchase in bulk then, while following list is by no means complete, it will help you get started in your search for aromatherapy suppliers. Check the Internet frequently to find new suppliers. Information for these companies was accurate when this book was published however, web sites and contact information may have changed or been deleted since publication.

The Aromatherapy Company

Web Site: http://www.thearomatherapycompany.co.nz/
E-Mail: website@starproducts.co.nz

PO Box 6615, Wellesley Street, 1141
Auckland
New Zealand

enquiries: phone 1800 104 029
orders: fax 1800 769 764
email: auorders@starproducts.co.nz

Description: The Aromatherapy Company was established in 1990 and has gone on to become a leading supplier of Home Fragrance and body care products. Kiwi ingenuity, combined with the consumers' desire for stronger, natural, pure products and environmental accountability from the corporate sector, has seen the Aromatherapy Company become a major force in the natural products market here in New Zealand and abroad.

Aura Cacia
Web Site: http://www.auracacia.com
E-Mail: customercare@auracacia.com
Telephone: (800) 437-3301
5398 31st Street
Urbana, IL 52345
Description: Aura Cacia sells a variety of essential oil related products
and high quality essential oils on line and wholesale to health food
store. The essential oils that you find in your local health food store are
most likely to Aura Cacia.

Birch Hill Happenings
Web Site: http://www.birchhillhappenings.com/aroma1.htm
E-Mail: albuddy1@aol.com
2898 County Road 103
Barnum, MN 55707-8808
Telephone: (218) 384-9294
Fax: (218) 384-3975
Description: Large selection of 100% Pure essential oils for therapeutic
aromatherapy. Also carrier oils, diffusers, charts, decoders, bottles,
unscented base products-shampoos, lotions & bath gels.

DHerb.Com
Website: http://dherbs.com
249 N Brand Blvd, Suite 518
Glendale, CA 91203
Toll Free: 818-396-4629
E-mail: info@trinityherb.com
Web site: www.trinity.com
DHerbs is a great wholesale source for essential oils in quantities from
1/3 oz to 16 ounces. They also wholesale bottles, bulk herbs and lots of
other interesting products.

Dr. Weed's Nature's Sunshine
Web Sites: http://www.mynsp.com/weed
               http://www.a-better-way.com
Email: Dr.Weed@a-better-way.com
Telephone: (314) 739-1492
Description: Dr. Weed is chiropractor, herbalist and acupuncturists,
and a Nature's Sunshine distributor. In addition to essential oils you
can order herbal supplements from him. He also has an on-line natural

health school that offers a basic natural health course at
http://www.naturalhealthschool.com   While there are lots of Nature's
Sunshine distributors around, Dr. Weed is the one that I use when I
need one.

EcoSevi

Web Site: http://www.ecosevi.com/
4401 Eastern Ave.
Box 26
Baltimore, Maryland 21224
Phone: 410.444.4461
Fax: 410.779.9105

Enfleurage

Web Site: http://www.enfleurage.com
E-Mail: oils@enfleurage.com
321 Bleecker Street
New York, NY 10014
Telephone: (888) 387-0300
Fax: (212) 337-0842
Description: Wholesale/retail. APP hydrosols, diffusers, aromatics from
around the world.

Frontier Natural Products Co-op

Web Site: http://www.frontiercoop.com/gsearch.php?s=essential+oil
E-Mail: customercare@frontiercoop.com
Frontier Natural Products Co-op
2990 Wilderness Place, Suite 200
Boulder, CO 80301
Telephone: (800) 786-1388
Description: Frontier Natural Products Co-op carries 100% pure
essential oils (many organic!), carrier oils and accessories. We have an
in-house Quality Assurance Lab which ensures all of our oils are pure
and of the highest quality available.

Nature's Gift Aromatherapy Products

Web Site: http://www.naturesgift.com
E-Mail: marge@naturesgift.com
1040 Cheyenne Blvd.
Madison, TN 37115

Telephone: (615) 612-4270
Fax: (615) 860-917
Description: they offer superb essential oils, sourced internationally, hydrosols, healing blends, aromatherapy accessories - diffusers, bottles, lamps, carrier oils.

Herbal Healer Academy

Web Sites: http://www.herbalhealer.com/
Email: HHA2012@aol.com
Telephone: 1- 870-269-5424
Address: HHA Inc., 127 McCain Drive, Mountain View, AR 72560
Description: Dr. McCain carries a large selection of essential oils, herbs, and herbal formulations. In addition the Herbal Healer Academy has an extensive offering of distance education courses.

Norfolk Essential Oils

Web Site: http://www.neoils.com
E-Mail: sales@neoils.demon.co.uk
Pates Farm, Tipsend, Welney
Wisbech, PE14 9SQ England
Telephone: 44(0)1354638065
Fax: 44(0)1354638149
Description: Growers and distillers of pure essential oils in England from crops grown on their own farms and distilled by steam.

One Planet

Web Site: http://www.oneplanetnatural.com
E-Mail: oneplanet@oneplanetnatural.com
157 Alabama Drive
Jacksonville, AR 72076
Toll-Free Telephone: (877) 754-0040
Description: Pure essential oils at very reasonable prices. FREE catalog and sample oils upon request. Secure online ordering. Major credit cards and checks. Our FYI section contains information on essential oil usage, descriptions, systems guide, and safety.

SunRose Aromatics

Web Site: http://www.sunrosearomatics.com
E-Mail: sunrose112@aol.com

P.O. Box 98
Throggs Neck Station
Bronx, NY 10465
Telephone: (718) 792-9451
Fax: (718) 792-9451
Description: Importers of essential oils from country of origin, wholesale/retail, no minimums, reasonable prices. Carrier Oils, Massage Blends, diffuser blends, diffusers, soaps.

.

PROFESSIONAL ASSOCIATIONS

United States

Alliance of International Aromatherapists
http://www.alliance-aromatherapists.org/

International Aromatherapy and Herb Association
www.aztecfreenet.org/makingscents/

National Association for Holistic Aromatherapy
www.naha.org

Aromatherapy Registration Council
www.aromatherapycouncil.org

International Aromatherapy Associations

Canada:

British Columbia Alliance of Aromatherapy
www.bcaoa.org

British Columbia Association of Practicing Aromatherapists
www.bcapa.org

Canadian Federation of Aromatherapists
www.cfacanada.com

Japan:

Japan Animal Aromatherapy Association
http://www.animalaromatherapy.jp/en-index.html

Korea:

Korean Aroma Society
http://www.aroma.or.kr/ (Note: This web site is in Korean)

New Zealand:

New Zealand Register of Holistic Aromatherapists
http://www.aromatherapy.org.nz/

United Kingdom:

Aromatherapy & Allied Practitioner's Association
www.aapa.org.uk

The Aromatherapy Council
www.aromatherapycouncil.org.uk/

International Federation of Professional Aromatherapists
www.ifparoma.org/

BOTTLES AND CONTAINERS

Our favorite supplier of bottles and containers are:

E. D. Luce Packaging

www.essentialsupplies.com

Creative Designs Enterprise
www.wholesalefragrances.com/

About the Authors

Heidi Murphy, M.Ed. is a professional counselor, mind-body expert and massage therapist. She has dedicated her life to the practice alternative holistic techniques and healing. She also works as a life coach. Heidi works closely with plants and flowers essences and implements them in her work with her clients. She spends her free time in nature learning more about the aromatherapy properties of flowers, the healing properties of medicinal herbs. To learn more about Heidi and her services email her at PeaceOfMindMurphy@gmail.com

Dr. Dave is a traditional naturopathic physician, master herbalist, advanced certified nutritional consultant and wellness coach. He has over 15 years of experience in the holistic healthcare field, including Ayurveda, nutritional and herbal consulting, aromatherapy, teaching stress reduction and Qi Gong, meditation, and healing techniques. He received his N.D. degree from the Trinity College of Natural Health, is board certified as an Alternative Medicine Practitioner by the American Alternative Medical Association, and earned a Certificate of Proficiency in Ayurvedic Medicine, with honors from the National Institute of Ayurvedic Medicine/Institute of Indian Medicine. His web site is http://www.compasswellnesscoaching.com.

INDEX

www.ingramcontent.com/pod-product-compliance
Lightning Source LLC
Chambersburg PA
CBHW070703290526
45790CB00001B/432